72240

	DATE DUE		

Sudden Death

and the

Myth of CPR

STEFAN TIMMERMANS

Foreword by

BERN SHEN, M.D.

TEMPLE UNIVERSITY PRESS
Philadelphia

Temple University Press, Philadelphia 19122

Copyright © 1999 by Temple University
All rights reserved
Published 1999
Printed in the United States of America

⊗ The paper used in this publication meets the requirements of the American National Standard for Information Sciences—Permanence of Paper for Printed Library Materials, ANSI Z39.48-1984

Library of Congress Cataloging-in-Publication Data

Timmermans, Stefan, 1968–
    Sudden death and the myth of CPR / Stefan Timmermans ; foreword by Bern Shen.
        p.   cm.
    Includes bibliographical references and index.
    ISBN 1-56639-715-4 (cloth : alk. paper). — ISBN 1-56639-716-2 (pbk. : alk. paper)
    1. CPR (First aid).   2. Cardiac arrest—Treatment.   3. Sudden death.   4. Emergency medical services—United States.   I. Title.
RC87.9.T56   1999
616.1'025—dc21   99-17282

In Memory of
   Moeke,
   Marthe,
   Ann

Contents

Foreword

The father of the bride entered our emergency department face up on a gurney, with one paramedic pumping on his chest and another squeezing oxygen into his lungs through an endotracheal tube. Although his perfectly shined shoes were still laced, his tuxedo had been carelessly torn open to make way for electrocardiographic electrodes, defibrillation pads, and IVs. Trailing him were his wife and son. He had been dead for 45 minutes, yet we stood poised in the resuscitation room, about to spend another hour trying to bring him back to life.

THIS BOOK examines a topic that has received surprisingly scant attention, despite the roughly 400,000 sudden deaths per year in the United States. How is it that a whole industry has grown up around cardiopulmonary resuscitation (CPR) when it seems to be so rarely successful? In exploring the answer, Stefan Timmermans meets the difficult challenge of articulating a common ground of interest for emergency medical staff, basic researchers, ethicists, sociologists, anthropologists, policy wonks, and that large and important constituency lumped under the inadequate rubric "lay readers."

Those who work in emergency medicine—first responders, paramedics, nurses, physicians, social workers, respiratory therapists, radiology techs, pharmacists, clergy, and others—will find, as I did, the full spectrum of emotional responses portrayed here, from a neophyte's unbridled enthusiasm to a veteran's more ambivalent stance. But the book goes beyond simple portrayal; it encourages us to examine our emotional responses in depth, a luxury we're rarely allowed during actual resuscitations.

Researchers and historians of medicine will appreciate Timmermans' detailed and careful outline of the evolution of CPR, which includes material from interviews with several of the field's leaders. Social scientists and health policy analysts will find a stimulating, somewhat contrary portrayal of what has become one of the pillars of Western biomedical practice, a portrayal in which Timmermans highlights the distinction between saving life and coping with death. Throughout the book, he disentangles and explores the complex knot of medical, social, and ethical issues with care and compassion.

The first three chapters provide an historical overview of social and medical attitudes toward dying, of the evolution of resuscitative techniques, and of the development of an emergency medicine infrastructure in the United States, including a widespread network of emergency transport and mass training of lay persons in basic life support. This overview sets the stage for the next three chapters, which summarize, with vivid vignettes, Timmermans' year-long ethnographic observations in two emergency departments. Along the way, Timmermans explicates social and emotional issues underlying CPR, such as patient and professional identity, the relationship between the rescuer and the rescued, the dynamics of the resuscitation team, the demystification of death for members of the resuscitation team, and the meanings of the CPR ritual. In addition, he analyzes decision making during resuscitations, including when to start and stop, and deciding—and decoding—when a person is dead and what makes for a "good," "bad," or "tragic" resuscitation. In the final chapter, Timmermans explores policy issues and potential nonbiomedical improvements to current CPR practice, such as allowing family members to be present during resuscitation efforts or paying more explicit attention to the needs of the survivors.

Readers will find that this book stimulates further biomedical, social, and ethical questions. In the biomedical sphere, how might medical research help CPR fulfill more of its historical promise? Perhaps detections of T-wave alternans or possibly beat-to-beat variability might lead to better prediction of susceptibility to sudden death. If we get better at predicting who might be at higher risk for sudden death, perhaps more patients will survive with intact neurological function. Are there opportunities for health care information technology to strengthen the "chain of survival"— for example, by automatic dispatch of medics or by more rapid retrieval of a patient's medical record?

In the social sphere, are there ways other than CPR to fulfill some of the nonmedical functions of seemingly futile resuscitations? For example, could public education possibly change societal attitudes toward death, or toward death in the home as opposed to death in the hospital? In what ways might sudden death and resuscitation be viewed differently in other cultures, both in the United States and abroad? And what about the experiences of the patients and their families? Unfortunately, constrained by the institutional review boards of the hospitals in which he did his observations, Timmermans was forced to focus on the experiences of the staff rather than of the patients.

In the ethical arena, a growing body of literature has developed around questions of what constitutes "futile" care, and the concept of a "good death." Are there ways to maximize the chance that a sudden death will be a good death? What are the pros and cons of trying to eliminate all disparities in how different patients are resuscitated? Are there ethical costs to the reification of CPR as a pillar of modern emergency medicine? What might be the consequences if managed care treatment protocols begin to specify when resuscitation efforts will and will not be reimbursed?

I feel triply implicated in this discussion of CPR: as an emergency physician with nearly two decades of prehospital and emergency department work, both in the United States and abroad; as a student of one of the pioneers of modern CPR—Dr. Peter Safar; and as the widower of a wife who was not, and could not have been, saved from a sudden death by resuscitative efforts. Like many readers, I've confronted the sudden death of individuals and its ripple effects on their families, caregivers, and the broader social network. As a physician, I've both rejoiced at "good saves" and felt disquiet at "failures" or, even worse, "bad saves," without fully being able to delineate crisply the boundaries of these categories. Perhaps for some readers, for Timmermans, and for myself, the loss of a loved one has raised important questions about our attitudes toward death and toward technologies designed to thwart it.

This book invites us to think more deeply about healing, even in the face of sudden death, and about resuscitation, not only of the patient but also of the survivors and caregivers. I hope this book will help all of us, including the family of the father of the bride, find some measure of wisdom and peace in our society's rituals surrounding CPR.

Bern Shen, M.D., M.Phil.
Clinical Assistant Professor, Emergency Medicine,
University of California, San Francisco
Research Scientist, Hewlett–Packard Labs, Palo Alto

Preface

THIS BOOK is for everyone who has taken a cardiopulmonary re-suscitation (CPR) course and wondered what would happen if he or she actually had to use CPR. Should you resuscitate or not? How likely are you to save a life? What happens if you don't save a life? Should you resuscitate even if is very unlikely that you will save a life? This book is also for the survivors of CPR, who are exceptionally lucky to have survived. I hope as well to provide answers to the many questions of bereaved relatives and friends who have been haunted by concerns about what went wrong when a loved one did not survive a resuscitative effort. In addition, this book is for the many health-care providers in emergency medicine who wonder how we can improve resuscitative care. I observed your resuscitative efforts and listened carefully to your stories of caring for people during sudden death. I hope that, after reading this book, you will be inspired to change resuscitative care in your departments. Finally, this book is for social scientists interested in the medicalization of sudden death.

At the core of this book is the paradox that people living in the United States and other Western societies resuscitate and keep resuscitating although these efforts rarely save lives. I explain the gap between the purpose of the technique and its actual result by looking at the development of resuscitation techniques and at the construction of an aggressive interventionist emergency system. After providing an overview of the historical and structural factors behind the current emergency medical infrastructure, I describe the emergency department, where most resuscitation efforts takes place, and I explain how professional staff make sense of routine resuscitation. This analysis points to the different purposes resuscitative efforts serve besides saving lives, and it identifies the problems with the current system of resuscitative care. In the end, my goal is to highlight ways to turn sudden death into a more compassionate and dignified passing.

I feel privileged to have received the support of many while researching and writing this book. Some people's contributions are especially visible. I am especially grateful to Leigh Star, Andy Pickering,

Norm Denzin, Peter Conrad, Marc Berg, Laura Neumann, Ruth Baxter, Debi Osnowitz, Michael Ames, my relatives in Belgium, and Anselm Strauss. Leigh generously offered me her mentorship throughout all the colorful tribulations of the research process and gently invited me to cross disciplinary boundaries. Andy pointed me to the "so what?" question. Norm encouraged me to leave the safe haven of classical ethnographic writing. Peter reminded me of a well-defined body of medical sociology. Marc kept me on my toes with his warm friendship, collaboration, and insightful remarks. Laura helped me transcribe some of the interviews and provided thoughtful comments on an earlier version of this book. Ruth convinced me that there is more to life and death than sociology and kept me smiling through the writing process. Debi offered a superb editing job. Mike was a patient critic and editor in the rewriting and publishing process. My relatives in Belgium encouraged me from a distance. Finally, I am grateful to the late Anselm Strauss, my academic "grandfather," whose theory, method, and friendly reminders permeate this work.

I am also much indebted to all the nurses, physicians, technicians, paramedics, respiratory therapists, social workers, and chaplains who allowed me to witness their lifesaving efforts and shared their stories in interviews. I especially want to thank "Ruth Berns" (all names of resuscitation staff and patients are pseudonyms), who, more than anyone else, shared her story and her friendship with me. For the historical part of this book, I am very grateful for the help of the archivists Crawford Keenan, Gerard Shorb, and Ms. Cavagnero at the Alan Mason Chesney Medical Archives of the Johns Hopkins Medical Institutions and for the help of the librarians of the medical library at the University of Illinois. I also would like to thank Drs. Bahnson, Isaacs, Jude, Safar, and Knickerbocker for sharing their views about the history of CPR.

Several people commented on at least one chapter of this book. I thank Amy Agigian, Madeleine Akrich, Renée Anspach, Amber Ault, Isabel Baszanger, Margaret Baxter, Oliver Benoit, Nancy Berns, Geof Bowker, Perry Bridger, Maryellen Burke, Monica Casper, Clifford Christians, Adele Clarke, Claire Cummings, Antoinette de Bont, Elaine Draper, Steven Epstein, Gary Alan Fine, the late Diana Forsythe, Joan Fujimura, Emilie Gomart, Judy Hanley, Karen Hansen, Joe Hopper, Niranjan Karnik, Susan Kahn, Christa Kelleher, John Kelly, Katrin Kriz, Sarah Lamb, Valerie Leiter, Tim Liao, John Lie, Mike Lynch, Evan Melhado, Madonna Harrington Meyer, Annemarie Mol, Jessica Muller,

Buddy Peshkin, Victoria Pitts, Jude Preissle, Eli Sagan, David Schwein-gruber, Steve Shapin, Maury Stein, Reya Stevens, Mindy Stombler, Veerle Stroobants, Kari Thoresen, Alexandra Todd, Jef Verhoeven, Paul Vernon, Kath Weston, Jack Whalen, Angela Yancik, and Barbara Zang.

I thank the Program of Ethics and Values at the University of Illinois for its financial support, the sociology department of the University of Illinois for the Geisert dissertation writing fellowship, and Brandeis University for the Mazer award to finish this book. Parts of Chapter 4 were published as "Saving Lives or Identities? The Double Dynamic of Technoscientific Scripts," in *Social Studies of Science* (1996) 26 (4): 769–99; an early version of Chapter 5 was published as "Social Death as a Self-Fulfilling Prophecy: David Sudnow's 'Passing On' Revisited," in *The Sociological Quarterly* (1998) 39 (3): 453–72; and a more elaborate version of Chapter 7 was published as "High Tech in High Touch: The Presence of Relatives and Friends During Resuscitative Efforts," in *Scholarly Inquiry for Nursing Practice* (1997) 11 (2): 152–67.

I dedicate this book to the memory of three strong women from three generations who all died in 1990–91, when I first began thinking about this project: my grandmother Augusta, or "Moeke," the warm center of the Timmermans family; my mother, Marthe, whom I probably resemble most; and my favorite cousin, Ann, for whom the technique I will follow in the next pages failed to fulfill its promise.

Sudden Death and the Myth of CPR

Introduction

What They Didn't Tell You in Your CPR Course

It is 9:35 on a Thursday evening in February. The weather forecast predicts sleet and maybe an ice storm. Ruth Berns,[1] an emergency department (ED) nurse, shivers when she pulls the curtain around a patient's bed. She thinks of her husband, a firefighter and avid motorcycle rider. "I hope he'll be safe tonight," she prays. When she walks back to the nursing station, she quickly glances at the patient board. With the weather forecast, this could be a busy night in the ED. Until now it has been rather quiet: a nursing-home patient's broken finger, a child with a sore throat, a regular patient with benign chest pain, two minor motor-vehicle accidents, and a woman who needs a rabies shot. Berns walks to the computer, orders the rabies vaccine, and prepares the five injections that precede it. While she calculates the exact dosage on the basis of the patient's weight, a radio call comes in. Lisa Lopez, her colleague, takes the call.

Shortly, Lopez comes over to Berns and says, "It was Bow ambulance. They have a code—a guy, 56 years old. Can you take him in room six?" When Berns nods, Lopez fills her in: "It was a witnessed arrest. They started CPR after about five minutes. Extensive cardiac history. The paramedics gave him epinephrine, lidocaine, shocked him at least four times. They should be here in about five minutes." Lopez then asks the department secretary to page the respiratory therapists, the nurse supervisor, and the social worker while she gives Dr. Michael Sears the same synopsis that she gave Berns. Berns motions Derrick Tovey, the ED technician, to follow her and tells him that a code is on the way. Together they ready the drugs and switch on the EKG monitor. The respiratory therapists, Lopez, and the nurse supervisor join them. They wait for the patient to arrive.

At 9:42 P.M., the paramedics wheel the stretcher into the resuscitation room. One of them is pushing an oxygen bag connected to a tube in the patient's mouth while the other steers the stretcher. A third person, wearing a sheriff's department T-shirt, stands on a bar under the

1

stretcher administering chest compressions. The patient is a middle-aged white man who seems to be wearing formal clothing. His shirt is torn open, and his tie has been cut loose. On his chest, three leads are connected to a portable defibrillator, which is placed on the stretcher between his legs. Quickly he is transferred from the stretcher to the ED bed. The respiratory therapists determine whether he is intubated correctly, detach the ventilation bag from the tubing, and attach the patient to their own oxygen and ventilation bag. At the same time, Tovey takes over the compressions. Berns checks the IV line established by the paramedics while she listens to their report.

Dr. Sears enters. He asks, "What do we have here?" The paramedic repeats: "We found him at the City Hotel. Full cardiac arrest. There was no ambulance available; firefighters got him first. After five minutes they started CPR. The firefighters shocked him seven times; we shocked him six times. We pumped him full of epinephrine. I think we gave him at least five and a couple of lidocaines, and he didn't respond. No pulse. He's had open-heart surgery." Berns tries to hook the patient up to the monitor in the room. She asks the team to stop the CPR. After a while, the monitor shows a very irregular rhythm; an occasional peak followed by a straight line.

Dr. Sears stares at the rhythm on the monitor. He says, "OK. We'll keep this nonsense up for ten minutes." One of the respiratory therapists repeats in disbelief, "Ten minutes?" She is new to the hospital. The doctor looks at her, annoyed, and gestures. "We have obviously already done everything: glucose, bicarb, epinephrine, defibrillation...." He then turns to the paramedics and says, "This man looks older than 50." The paramedic answers, "He's actually 71 years old. He's from out of town. He was a speaker at the City Hotel."

The respiratory therapists seem to have a problem. It appears the air is not going directly from their oxygen bag into the patient's tube. They argue about a possible leak. They pull and turn the tube and replace a piece. Berns asks Dr. Sears, "Do we need to give him anything?" "Yes, give him another epi," Sears answers. The second technician puts a blood-pressure cuff around the glucose bag to squeeze out the last drips. Dr. Sears leaves the room.

After the first rush, things become a little quieter. The paramedic walks to the nurse supervisor, who is taking notes, and tells her in detail what he administered to the patient on the way to the hospital. With some difficulty, Berns has been able to put the epinephrine in the IV line.

She starts talking about another case, in which the nurses in a nursing home thought that a patient had had a seizure, "He wasn't breathing anymore. He was blue for the last five minutes." She adds sarcastically, "They were so happy that the paramedics were there." The listeners shake their head in disbelief. Berns adds, "We got him back two times with bicarb, just enough to let him die in intensive care."

Everyone is now waiting out the time. One of the respiratory therapists mentions a cousin who was in his thirties when he was found slumped over in his truck. The technician asks what happened. "They think he had a cardiac arrest in an asthma attack, but I don't know. I know he was severely asthmatic. He had two children and a third on the way." The glucose bag is almost empty, and Derrick asks whether they should replace it. "No," answers Lopez. "It's only three more minutes, and the family will be charged enough." Tovey stops the compressions for a couple of seconds to check the monitor again, but there is no change.

Dr. Sears returns with the social worker and asks, "Any change after the epi?" He answers himself, "He's not responding to anything, is he?" The paramedic walks in to pick up the portable defibrillator and comments that the patient was at the City Hotel to be awarded Farmer of the Year. The nurses look at the patient and sigh. Observing the ripped clothes hanging off the patient, Derrick observes, "This was probably his only good suit." Lopez turns to the social worker. "What's his name?" she asks. "Richard Elmer" is the response. The technician wonders, "Did you know that he had a cousin with him?" The social worker answers, "There's a whole family over there. Two daughters and he lost his wife in September...." Ruth Berns interrupts, "Stop. I don't want to know anymore. I already start crying when I watch the Oprah show. Today they had two quadriplegics who married after their spouses left them, and they focused for what seemed like an hour on how they tried to put their rings on each other's fingers. I just had to leave the room." The physician is amused by the marriage of quadriplegics. He bends over the patient to look at the monitor and says, "I'm going to declare this patient dead." "Okay" says the nurse supervisor, "It's 9:56." "Make it 9:55. That's easier to remember." replies the doctor. The cardiac rhythm is still as irregular as it was when the patient entered. Most people leave. Berns waits to take a printout of the EKG monitor. She needs a straight line. Then she gently pushes with her thumbs on Richard Elmer's eyelids to keep them down.

THE MYTH OF CPR

Richard Elmer collapsed. His pulse and breathing disappeared. Not so long ago, this would have been the moment of his death. His relatives, friends, and colleagues might have reflected on the irony that he died at a banquet held in his honor, and they would have mourned his sudden passing. But at his collapse, Elmer was not immediately—or, at least, not officially—dead, and his relatives undertook some very specific actions to keep him alive. They dialed 911, extended his neck, and placed their mouths on his mouth and their hands on his chest. By performing these simple steps, they set into motion a vast emergency system aimed at reversing the dying process. Similar scenarios are played out daily, hundreds of times throughout the country, underscoring resuscitation as the routine response to sudden death.

The most striking aspect of Elmer's story is its outcome. The resuscitative efforts of first responders, paramedics, and an entire ED armed with drugs and defibrillators were insufficient to keep him alive. Few people know that death is by far the most common outcome of out-of-hospital cardiopulmonary resuscitation (CPR) and the advanced cardiac life-support (ACLS) protocols used in the ED. Survival rates for out-of-hospital resuscitative efforts are hard to come by, and estimates vary widely, but there now exists some consensus. In a document approved by the American Heart Association, medical researchers ask,

> What is the maximum practical survival rate? The number of people resuscitated from sudden death by emergency personnel is not known. Nor is it known how many people can be resuscitated with a reasonable chance of surviving and remaining neurologically intact.... Though no national averages are available on the proportion of people who survive out-of-hospital cardiac arrests, *current estimates suggest that no more than 1–3% of victims live to be discharged from the hospital. The true percentage is probably even less.*[2]

These low percentages mean that in the overwhelming majority of resuscitative efforts,[3] people die. Still, we keep teaching schoolchildren CPR; we portray overwhelmingly successful resuscitative attempts on TV; and we invest millions of dollars in a sprawling emergency-system infrastructure to create the expectation that with resuscitative care every death may be averted. The widespread use and availability of resuscitation techniques in American society means that sudden death equals premature death, a death that by definition comes too early. People act as if death caused by heart attacks, strokes, and accidents is a treatable event, to be cured like a Strep throat infection with the right medical intervention. But if the purpose and expectation of CPR is to save human lives from sudden death, resuscitative interventions are largely failures. Their intended goal is rarely attained. Belief in resuscitation has the value of a revered cultural myth perpetuated by "real-life" television shows and the organizations promoting CPR. The techniques spin a tale of heroism, medical magic to overcome the adversity of death, and the holy grail of a prolonged life in everyone's reach. Unfortunately, the tale unravels—humans remain mortals—and the promise of saved lives remains mostly unfulfilled.

Even if very few lives are saved, the overuse of resuscitation defines people's experience with sudden death. For Richard Elmer's relatives, the outcome means the life or death of their loved one. For them, the resuscitative effort is a dramatic event. They did what they were supposed to do: they followed the CPR protocols, called 911, and saw how the paramedics transported Elmer to one of the best hospitals in the area. They rushed behind the ambulance, then waited in the ED's counseling room with a social worker. They told the social worker that Elmer had had heart problems, and the social worker explained to them that things did not look good. Still, family members were unprepared for the shock when Dr. Sears came into the room to inform them that Richard Elmer had died. Instead of dying among friends and relatives, Elmer died in the hospital among health-care personnel.

For the resuscitation team in the ED, the same reviving effort was a routine procedure. They did not expect the resuscitative effort to succeed in saving a life, but they still needed to continue resuscitating. There is an unspoken subtext in the attempt to revive Elmer to which only ED insiders are privy. The physician who considers the reviving procedure "nonsense" and his annoyance with the inexperienced respiratory therapist who expresses surprise at its duration, as well as the team's casual conversation about television shows, stories about other failed attempts, nonchalance about the time of death, and jokes about the ineffectiveness of CPR, all indicate that this resuscitative procedure is little more than a matter of going through the motions. Although health-care providers know that resuscitating is often futile, they continue the procedure because they perceive pressure from outside the ED.

Resuscitation also defines sudden death on a broader cultural level. These interventions indicate more than anything else how people in

Western societies at the turn of the twenty-first century have turned away from personal, community-centered dying and embarked instead on an elusive search for the postponement of death. Instead of passing away among relatives and friends with whom we have shared long histories, we pay white-coated professionals to deal with the sudden-dying process. Their work is secluded behind closed doors, and their task is to keep death at bay. With resuscitation protocols spelling out the script during the last moments, death becomes the wrong outcome. When the doors open, a cold body reappears in its finality, cleaned and arranged. The dying process remains invisible, and the customary phrase, "We did everything we could, but...." once again underscores that death should not have occurred. A society that builds and supports an extensive resuscitative system opts for aggressive intervention, death defiance, and medicalization of the dying process.

How Dignified Is Sudden Death?

The observation that resuscitative efforts save lives only rarely raises the issue of the quality of such a dying process. If a person who was supposed to keep living dies at the end of a resuscitative attempt, how socially meaningful is that dying? How dignified was Richard Elmer's death? If Elmer had been diagnosed with an aggressive, terminal cancer six months earlier, he would have had the opportunity to reflect on his impending end. He could have chosen to put closure on some aspects of his life, and—if he had the resources—he, his relatives, and his friends could have opted during the last weeks for different forms of palliative or hospice care, or they might even have considered assisted suicide. But unlike expected, lingering deaths, in which all parties have days, even months, to reflect on a course of action, the possibility of turning sudden death into a "good" parting moment seems to be severely limited because time, access, and resources are lacking. In addition, the very use of resuscitation techniques focuses on an attempt at reviving, not a consideration of impending death. Thus, while most patients are deceased at the end of resuscitative efforts, their loved ones are unprepared. At the last moments, resuscitative techniques have intervened.

In different ways, Elisabeth Kübler-Ross and the death-awareness movement, Dame Cicely Saunders and the hospice movement, Jack Kevorkian and physician-assisted suicide, and the Hemlock Society advocate dignified dying at the end of an expected lingering-illness trajectory. These advocates have championed alternatives to customary hospital practice. But who writes about, speaks for, or wants to change sudden death? This book examines the quality of sudden death at the end of resuscitative efforts. As a sociologist, my purpose is to analyze how people use resuscitative techniques to make sense of sudden death. I therefore will investigate out-of-hospital resuscitative practice not as a set of interventions to save lives (which rarely happens anyway) but as a medical action that frames the dying experience. My investigation concentrates on the organization and actual experience of resuscitating in EDs. Like the neonatal intensive-care observer Renée Anspach, I am more interested in how decisions about life and death are made than about how they should be made.[4] My approach differs from the concerns of ethicists, who often use idealistic, extreme resuscitative scenarios to debate morally sound decision-making. I also diverge from legal scholars, who examine the legal ramifications of the decision to resuscitate or withhold resuscitative care. Finally, I differ from emergency physicians and researchers who have written extensively about improving survival rates by changing the emergency-care system, resuscitative protocols, or clinical decision-making. All these analysts provide recommendations about how or when one should resuscitate, but they are less concerned with how resuscitative care is accomplished in practice. Most also assume that the quick and proper use of resuscitative techniques regularly leads to saved lives.

If we want to understand how resuscitative technology might provide meaning to sudden death, we need to withhold judgment about these techniques. Ethicists and many social scientists often refer to resuscitative technology as an example of an excessively technology-driven medicine. They repeat the argument that advanced medical technology has corrupted the dying experience, making it somehow less "natural" (see Chapter 1). At the same time, physicians and some ethicists hail the same technology for saving lives that would otherwise be lost. This blame–hail reasoning isolates medical technology and ascribes to it too much power. In line with a recent wave of science and technology studies, I believe that the important task is to follow technology in action and show how it generates new meanings and changes our understanding about the finality of life.[5] Such an approach does not imply an uncritical stance, but, as I show, it ultimately can be directed toward evaluating the technology and improving the dying experience.

I address the dignity of sudden dying with a combination of historical material, observations, and interviews. In the historical chapters, I explore how, in one generation, American society invested heavily in an emergency medical system and fostered the belief that every sudden death is potentially reversible. Relying on primary archival sources and published medical studies, the historical chapters document the growing medicalization of sudden death, the "statisticulation" (Darrell Huff's term for the manipulation of people by the use of statistical material[6]) used by emergency-system policymakers, and the neglect of sudden death by the death-awareness community. The result is a vast emergency infrastructure centered on universally used resuscitation techniques that potentially enroll every American as a first responder and potential victim in the resuscitation project.

In the ethnographic chapters, I look at what it means to resuscitate on a daily basis when almost no one survives. Using interviews with forty-five ED staff and fourteen months of observations of out-of-hospital resuscitative efforts in two EDs in a Midwestern town (see Appendix), I map how the staff balances social and clinical patient characteristics to reach the "right" decision about life and death during a resuscitative effort. In addition, I explore how a health-care novice learns to evaluate a resuscitative effort on grounds other than its outcome. In the last chapter, I describe some possible avenues for change that would prepare people for impending death. Specifically, while the patient is hanging between life and death, relatives and friends could be given the opportunity to say goodbye to their loved one and be part of these very important last moments. For example, instead of discussing talk shows at the end of the resuscitative effort, a social worker or chaplain could have accompanied two of Richard Elmer's closest relatives into the resuscitation room. There they could have said the last things they regretted never having said; they could have touched his forehead or just witnessed with their own eyes the final moments of his life. In that case, a resuscitative effort would have been not only a lifesaving attempt but also a unique occasion to face the impending death and begin the mourning process. It would have become a parting ritual not in spite of, but because of, the available technology.

As an example of what could be retrieved with some adaptations in current resuscitative practice, I would like to contrast Richard Elmer's death to the anthropologist Barbara Myerhoff's account of the sudden death of a popular Jewish community leader and teacher, Jacob Koved, at a party in honor of his ninety-fifth birthday.[9] Although firefighters transported Koved to the hospital, his friends and family resisted the interpretation that he did not die among them and dismissed the importance of the last-ditch reviving effort. After Koved was transferred to the hospital, a rabbi took center stage and spoke:

> We have had the honor of watching a circle come to its fullness and close as we rejoiced together. We have shared Jacob's wisdom and warmth and though the ways of God are mysterious, there is meaning in what happened today. I was with Jacob backstage and tried to administer external heart massage. In those few moments with him behind the curtain, I felt his strength. There was an electricity about him, but it was peaceful and I was filled with awe. When the firemen burst in, it felt wrong because they were big and forceful and Jacob was gentle and resolute. He was still directing his life, and he directed his death. We will say Kaddish, the mourner's prayer.

Myerhoff observed:

> People shuffled towards the stage, talking quietly in Yiddish. Many crossed the room to embrace friends. Among the old people, physical contact was usually very restrained, yet here they eagerly sought each other's arms. Several wept softly. As dictated by Jewish custom, no one approached the family, but only nodded to them as they left. There were many such spontaneous expressions of traditional Jewish mourning customs, performed individually, with the collective effect of transforming the celebration into a commemoration. Olga reached down and pulled out the hem of her dress, honoring the custom of rending one's garments on news of a death. Someone had draped her scarf over the mirror in the women's room as tradition required. Moshe poured his glass of tea into a saucer. Finally, the Center had emptied. People clustered together on the benches outside to continue talking and reviewing the events of the afternoon. Before long, all were in agreement that Jacob had certainly died among them. The call to the rescue squad was a formality, they agreed. Said Moshe, "You see, it is the Jewish way to die in your community. In the old days, it was an honor to wash the body of the dead. No one went away and died with strangers in a hospital. The finest people dressed the corpse and no one left him alone for a minute. So Jacob died like a good Yid. Not everybody is so lucky."

If we compare Richard Elmer's death with the death of Jacob Koved, the similarity is that neither could just die. Even a ninety-five-year-old man needed to be resuscitated. The difference is that in Koved's situation, the resuscitative attempt was secondary to the community mourning. Koved's death was socially meaningful in spite of the reviving attempt. In Elmer's case, the resuscitative interventions prevailed, and the medical goal of saving a life overshadowed his passing. Elmer's relatives and friends were pushed aside by the paramedics and left in a counseling room in the ED. They left Elmer when he was somewhere in limbo between life and death, and when they saw him again, he was officially dead.

We need not fall back on the mourning rituals of a Jewish immigrant community to make sudden death meaningful. There are other ways to adapt the use of resuscitative interventions to the needs of relatives, friends, and all of us to put closure on sudden death. Resuscitative procedures rarely save lives, but with some modifications, we may be able to save sudden death.

1   Death Awareness in the United States

IN HER best-selling books, Elisabeth Kübler-Ross crystallized an emerging recognition in the late sixties that something had gone profoundly wrong with the way people died. She and other researchers noted that death had become a taboo topic in Western cultures and that the dying experience lacked the significance it once had. Over time, the perceived "good" community death had disappeared and had been replaced with a depersonalized, anxiety-filled hospital passing. Instead of integrating death into everyday life, Americans had expelled the dying to hospitals, where they hoped for a quick medical fix. In response, health-care professionals, scholars from a variety of disciplines, and informed people united in a social movement[1] to change the problems associated with dying.

The resuscitation pioneer Claude Beck and his assistant David Leighlinger agreed in 1962 that something was profoundly wrong with death and dying. People indeed feared death. Life was a sanctuary, and once the sanctuary was threatened, people became paralyzed with fear. Few knew how to react, and hesitation in crisis could cause death. According to Beck, "some hearts are too good to die" and "death can be reversed in these good hearts." Beck therefore argued for the dissemination of one of his inventions, the electrical defibrillator, to reverse the dying process.

In their different ways, Beck and Kübler-Ross were visionaries who wanted to change the way people die. Kübler-Ross spearheaded a social movement to make death more dignified while Beck promoted extensive medical efforts to reverse the dying process with resuscitation techniques. These separate movements help to explain how we now think about sudden death. We approach sudden death not as an event that needs to become more dignified but as "premature" death, a death that could have been avoided if we were able to apply the right technology quickly enough. The result is a two-tiered dying system. At the end of a lingering chronic-illness trajectory, the dying person and caretakers have some choices about the last days or months of life. Sudden death, in contrast, is an event securely controlled by medical professionals.

THE EMERGENCE OF DEATH AWARENESS

When American social researchers began to consider dying in the mid-sixties, the face of the dying person and the place of death had changed dramatically. Since the turn of the century, few people had personally witnessed other people's deaths. Declining fertility and, to a lesser extent, declining mortality rates had increased both the proportion and the absolute numbers of people living longer. Between 1900 and 1960, the mortality rate had dropped from 17.2 per 1,000 to 9.5 per 1,000, while the infant-mortality rate kept dropping even more, from 47 per 1,000 infants in 1940 to 26 per 1,000 in 1960. Death was largely a phenomenon of the elderly. Public-health and medical measures had also produced a shift in common causes of death. Deaths from infectious diseases among the frail gave way to deaths caused by heart disease and strokes. The death rate from tuberculosis, for example, declined from a level of 184.8 per 100,000 in 1900 to 4.1 per 100,000 in 1965. Over the same interval, typhoid fever, diphtheria, and whooping cough were virtually eliminated. On the other hand, the death rate from heart disease rose from 359.2 per 100,000 in 1900 to 518.2 per 100,000 in 1965.[2]

In the first half of the twentieth century, hospitals ceased to be poorhouses and instead became places for caring, curing, and ultimately dying. The number of hospitals in the United States expanded from fewer than two hundred in 1873 to 4,438 in 1928, 5,237 in 1955, and 5,736 in 1965.[3] Hospitals and long-term–care institutions replaced the home as the place in which increasing numbers of Americans spent the last days of their lives. At the turn of the century, only 15 to 20 percent of people died in hospitals. By 1949, these institutions were the sites of 50 percent of American deaths; by 1977, more than 70 percent of Americans died in hospitals. In addition, the dying process became longer, punctuated with multiple hospitalizations. Within hospitals—especially teaching hospitals—the priority of prolonging life emerged against the background of medical-practice innovations. Hospital personnel warned patients that "once you come to the hospital, you ought to know that everyone is concerned to preserve your life. The person has no choice"[4] in the matter.

Demographic changes and the rise of hospitals took place over a number of decades, and not until the sixties were these changes considered problematic, a part of a growing cultural disappointment with the established institutions, including medicine. The catalyzing event was the U.S. involvement in the Vietnam war. Much earlier, in the aftermath of the First World War, Sigmund Freud[5] had argued that wars obliterate our customary denial of death and press upon us a heightened sense of mortality. The Vietnam war was the first televised war; its battlefield news coverage brought images of abruptly curtailed young lives in body bags. Death became imprinted on the nation's consciousness, and the shockwaves did more than increase death awareness; they rippled into a general cultural malaise. Where the Second World War—believed to have been won through the concerted efforts of scientists and the military[6]—promised modernism, optimism, and progress, the Vietnam war generated a sense of disillusionment and vulnerability. New doubts suggested that "authorities can be wrong,"[7] and widespread introspection about the use and abuse of power extended to religion, the family, the state, the military, and medicine.

In this general climate of questioning authority, the way people died was examined critically and found wanting. When Kübler-Ross visited and interviewed dying patients, death had become an "unavoidable reality" that was still much avoided. In the late sixties, scholars and literary critics discussed how an entire culture was in a state of "denial" about the possibility of death. Geoffrey Gorer first pointed out the "taboo" of dying in his essay, "The Pornography of Death."[8] He argued that after the First World War, society had refused to address personal death and instead became obsessed with the "pornographic" representation of a depersonalized and abstract death in the media. We had become death voyeurs, fascinated with the gore of violent death while simultaneously ignoring the possibility of our own personal death. Dying had received an unreal character; it occurred in the abstract, but not to us. Other works echoed this message: Herman Feifel's influential edited volume *The Meaning of Death* characterized American society by a deep "denial and avoidance of the countenance of death."[9]

From a historical point of view, Philippe Ariès was instrumental in documenting the impoverishment and unnaturalness of contemporary modern dying. Although Ariès's writings were published later, they resonated with the emerging death-awareness movement. In his classics *Western Attitudes Towards Death and Dying*[10] and *The Hour of Our Death*,[11] Ariès chronicled death rites and customs of the past centuries. The old model for dying was what Aries labeled "the tame death." This pre–Victorian deathbed scene was not a death that would become domesticated over time but one that had been tame and had now become wild (i.e., fearful, denied, lonely, and dirty):

In the early twentieth century, before World War I, throughout the Western world of Latin culture, be it Catholic or Protestant, the death of a man [*sic*] still solemnly altered the space and time of a social group that could be extended to include the entire community. The shutters were closed in the bedroom of the dying man, candles were lit, holy water was sprinkled; the house filled with grave and whispering neighbors, relatives and friends. At the church, the passing bell tolled and the little procession left carrying the *Corpus Christi*.

After death, a notice of bereavement was posted on the door (in lieu of the old abandoned custom of exhibiting the body or the coffin by the door of the house). All the doors and windows of the house were closed except the front door, which was left ajar to admit everyone who was obliged by friendship or good manners to make a final visit. The service at the church brought the whole community together, including latecomers who waited for the end of the funeral to come forward; and after the long line of people had expressed their sympathy to the family, a slow procession, saluted by passersby, accompanied the coffin to the cemetery. And that was not all. The period of mourning was filled with visits: visits of the family to the cemetery and visits of relatives and friends to the family.

Then, little by little, life returned to normal, and there remained only the periodic visits to the cemetery. The social group had been stricken by death, and it had reacted collectively, starting with the immediate family and extending to a wider circle of relatives and acquaintances.[12]

Ariès considered this community-centered death the historic ideal. Over time, however, changes had occurred in the way people died. Although death had long remained a public event, Ariès explained, a more rapid and strong tendency to isolate death and dying in the Western world had begun in the nineteenth century. The isolation of death was closely linked to the rise of medicine as a science and a profession.[13] Nineteenth-century physicians complained about the presence of neighbors and friends at the dying hour, and death became reserved for the close relatives. Invasive medical procedures performed as a last resort required the relocation of the dying body to the hospital. These were the first steps in the gradual medicalization, commercialization, and technology dependence of dying.[14] The final result was an isolated, private, anonymous death in a hospital room where the dying person was surrounded by strangers.[15] Dying had become a "dirty" event while funeral and mourning practices disappeared or became discrete. Ariès lamented the secularization and individualization of the pre–Victorian dying ritual and the erosion of the art of dying, the *ars moriendi*. In Ariès' opinion, American dying in the sixties was the low point in the history of the denial of death.

As historical studies offered an idealized pre-Victorian deathbed scene as a model of meaningful dying, they also set the terms of comparison for dying in modern society. More than anyone else, Kübler-Ross captured the public's imagination as she alerted people to the gap between the "social" death of the past and the predicament of dying in the present. In her best-selling book, *On Death and Dying*, she observed how patients are abandoned by relatives and health-care professionals when they are seriously ill and dying. Instead of ignoring dying patients, Kübler-Ross gave them the opportunity to express their thoughts and feelings in a psychiatric interview. On the basis of the stories she heard, Kübler-Ross divided the dying process into five stages: denial and isolation; anger and resentment; bargaining and an attempt to postpone death; depression and a sense of loss; and acceptance. She emphasized the importance of maintaining hope for psychological well-being. She argued for reuniting dying patients with their families and friends, for talking about and accepting impending death. Her books "launched her on a perpetual round of house calls to dying patients and their families, and a continuous cycle of public lectures and 'Life, Death and Transition Workshops' attended by hundreds of persons."[16]

Over the years, several scholars have criticized Kübler-Ross's stage model—especially the normative implications of accepting one's impending death and the religious undertones of her interpretations—and, later, her unwavering belief in near-death experiences, life after death, communication with spirits, and cosmic consciousness.[17] Although the specifics of Kübler-Ross's theory are now largely discredited, there is no doubt about her role as a pioneer and charismatic leader when she sensitized people in the late sixties and early seventies to the problems with the modern ways of dying.

While psychologists studied the emotional vacuum surrounding death, sociologists provided empirical studies that painted an even grimmer picture. Structural and cultural factors isolated the dying. Sociologists argued not that the United States was a death-denying society, but that the environment in which death occurred fostered denial.[18] For example, Barney Glaser and Anselm Strauss[19] conducted a study of death and dying in hospitals of the San Francisco Bay area. There they noted that patients were abandoned by staff once a chronic condition entered the terminal stages. Faced with physicians convinced that they knew what was "best" for their patients, terminally ill patients had difficulty obtaining an honest assessment of their condition. Physicians would keep terminal patients in a "closed awareness context" about their fatal diagnosis and terminal prognosis. The result was that the staff engaged in a complex interactional game of hiding signs, thwarting and dismissing suspicions, and conspiring with relatives—all in an effort to avoid informing the patient. A patient who found out anyway was not necessarily in an improved position, because such a patient might enter an even more isolating context of "mutual pretense" in which everyone knew the terminal prognosis but no one was willing even to mention it.

Simone de Beauvoir provided an example of such a death when she described the last month of her mother's life in 1963. A surgeon cajoled the de Beauvoir sisters to lie to their mother and tell her that an operation was for peritonitis instead of a virulent and widely spread cancer. One sister asked the doctor, "But what shall we say to Maman when the disease starts again, in another place?" "Don't worry about that," the doctor responded. "We shall find something to say. We always do. And the patient always believes it."[20] No one explained that the mother was dying, but she knew that her end was near. When Simone de Beauvoir sorted through the suitcase she had brought home from the clinic after her mother passed away, she found a note directed to the sisters: "I should like a very simple funeral. No flowers or wreaths. But a great many prayers."[21] Thus, unless someone broke down and explicitly discussed the impending death, patients would die seemingly ignorant about what was happening but actually knowing what was awaiting them. Dying was a poignantly lonely and miserable event, clouded in feelings of betrayal and shame.

David Sudnow[22] offered the most damaging picture of dying in the sixties. He graphically depicted the alienation of death and dying in an ethnography of two hospitals. There he described how people who were still biologically alive were treated as if death had already occurred. Sudnow depicted a nurse who closed the eyelids of a dying patient before biological death had set in and student doctors who practiced intubation on fresh corpses. According to Sudnow's observations, people with a presumed low social value were treated less aggressively than those with a presumed high social value. Social status became a predictor for biological viability. (I revisit this critique in Chapter 5.) Sudnow also noted that relatives were discouraged from spending time with the deceased because such episodes interfered with the hospital's routines.

To complete the picture of the dying experience in the sixties, the investigative journalist Jessica Mitford critically analyzed the practices of the funeral industry in her widely read book *The American Way of Death*.[23] She charged that the funeral business was excessively commercial and took advantage of the emotional turmoil caused by the death of a loved one. Mitford described American funeral practices as overly lavish and expensive. The costly make-up, lining of the casket, and euphemisms used in the funeral industry promoted an image of life rather than death. Here, too, death was denied for the illusion of eternal life.

The books by Kübler-Ross, Glaser and Strauss, Ariès, and Mitford were widely read and resonated with the death experiences of a general public becoming attuned to the "plight of the dying" and searching for ways to turn the dying process into a dignified passing. "As the death with dignity movement's cause became popular in the 1960s and 1970s, groups assembled in hospitals, parishes, and colleges to talk about ways to change social conditions. Assemblies such as these served to reinforce participants' belief that something was wrong with the way the dying were treated and that social reform was required."[24] An early hospice organizer explained, "We were all just mad. We sat in my living room ... like hours. We all had some horror story. We were angry at the doctor, the nurse, someone. After a while we realized that our loved one might have received better care if he was at home. It was the place of care that caused the problem."[25] The growing public awareness was epitomized by the Special Committee on Aging of the U.S. Senate hearing on "Death with Dignity" in August 1972.[26] Specialized journals emerged around death and dying,[27] and university professors taught classes on the institutionalization of death.[28]

At the roots of the death-and-dying problem in the sixties lay an endemic cultural reluctance to face impending death. Lynn Lofland noted with exasperation that "the assertion that death is a taboo topic in America has been repeated so often, by so many people, in so many contexts, that one begins to believe it must surely, somewhere, be engraved on stone—the revealed words of the gods."[29] The modern dying experience had become a social problem, one that might be addressed like other social problems of the time: through a social movement. The emerging death-awareness movement dovetailed with other social movements, such as peace, civil rights, feminist and gay rights, home birthing, women's health, and other patient empowerment groups.[30] A patchwork of local and national initiatives tackled the problems of the dying experience. The social worker Phyllis Silverman, for example, advocated a de-medicalization of the grieving process and started the widow-to-widow project at Harvard Medical School in 1967. Patient and women's health advocates fought for the right of access to information to reach informed decisions. In medical curricula, educators and psychologists taught medical students how to break "bad" news to patients.[31] People also organized in buyers' clubs to purchase their own caskets in an attempt to bypass the funeral industry.

More radical activists proposed legal solutions to undignified dying. Increasingly, groups introduced right-to-die bills, although these bills faced great resistance from pro-life activists, who made abortion and euthanasia their two rallying points. Eventually, an unofficial alliance among church officials, right-to-life advocates, and death-with-dignity supporters focused on an organized approach to care for the terminally ill. This alliance promoted the concept of hospice as a method of care for the dying that involved traditional health-care providers but also gave the relatives and patients some choice in the continuation of medical intervention. Hospice rejected any talk about euthanasia. As hospice care became the major avenue for change, the general unease with dying became more specific.

HOSPICE CARE

The main alternative to traditional modern hospital dying emerged when leaders of a growing death-awareness movement infused the notion of hospice with more advanced ideas of palliative care. Hospices had existed since Greek and Roman times.[32] The predecessors of the most recent hospice wave came in 1879, when Sister Mary Aitkinhead opened Pure Lady's Hospice in Dublin, expressing her view that death was part of an eternal journey. By 1905, a similar facility, St. Joseph's Hospice, was established in London, and a medical officer introduced pain control as a central goal for hospice care. Subsequently, Dr. Cicely Saunders founded St. Christopher's Hospice in London, which has served as an inspiration and model for U.S. hospices. Touched by the predicament of a dying patient, Saunders wanted to ease the pain of cancer patients. Combining the roles of nurse, chaplain, and physician, she trained in pain management and symptom control and developed a terminal-care program that paid careful attention to positioning of the patient, dietary preferences, and massage. On her first visit to the United

States in 1963, she showed slides of cancer patients before and after they had received hospice treatment. The after-care patients seemed in much higher spirits, and their previously debilitating symptoms seemed under control. Saunders particularly impressed health-care workers concerned with care given to dying patients.[33] In 1966, Saunders visited the United States for a second time. During a stop at Yale University, she joined forces with Kübler-Ross,[34] who saw Saunders's hospice program as an institutional vehicle to implement her ideas for more humane dying.

In 1974, Connecticut Hospice in New Haven became the first full-service home-hospice program of its type in the United States, and by 1995 more than 2,000 hospice programs existed in the United States,[35] where hospice covers diverse initiatives: free-standing in-patient services, roving hospice teams, home-health agencies, and hospice services in hospitals. The prerequisite for these services is that the patient be at a stage of illness at which a cure can no longer be expected. Hospice care differs from traditional care in that the goal is no longer to cure the patient. This care is palliative: enhancing comfort through pain management; treating symptoms; and reducing anxiety, fear, and suffering. Relatives and other people important in the patient's life are part of the caregiving. Although hospice takes care of the dying, the emphasis is on living remaining life as fully as possible. Care is personal, low-technology, and aimed at re-creating the home instead of a hospital setting.

How does hospice care work? In 1990, Hamilton and Reid[36] published a detailed case history of Mary, a patient at the Hospice Care Service of Montreal's Royal Victoria Hospital. The 47-year-old Mary had undergone a radical mastectomy, chemotherapy, and radiation for breast cancer. These treatments had not stopped the cancer, which had spread to her lungs and bones. Although she could not work and suffered from severe shortness of breath, Mary preferred to stay at home with her husband, John, and 17-year-old daughter, Lucy. Her 21-year-old son, Henry, was away at school. Mary worried about her children, who were not told how serious her situation was. The visiting nurse from the palliative-care unit taught John and relatives how to provide good skin care. The nurse further contributed to Mary's physical care by discussing her condition with radiologists and other specialists and arranging for volunteers to transport Mary to outpatient hospital checkups. A physiotherapist taught her breathing exercises. The care was aimed at giving Mary a sense of control over her situation. In addition, the nurse addressed the needs of relatives. She convinced Mary and John to discuss the seriousness of the situation with their children, and when Henry withdrew from the family, she encouraged him to talk to his mom. The nurse also addressed Mary's overall quality of life when she helped Mary to make a turban and provided her with a wig when she was distressed about her hair loss. When the situation worsened, Mary was transported to the in-hospital palliative-care unit, where she died three days later. The home-care nurse remained involved in the final care.

Mary's hospice care addressed her own physical needs and emotional distresses as well as the fears and questions of her close relatives. But even under ideal circumstances, hospice is not for everyone. Cancer patients are typical hospice clients. To qualify for hospice care, the patient needs to acknowledge impending death; the set-up thus works better for patients suffering from lingering illnesses such as AIDS and cancer. For this reason, sudden death does not fit the hospice philosophy and institutions.[37] People who die suddenly do not have the opportunity and time to address spiritual and social questions at the end of life. Hard-core advocates of the hospice death consider sudden death too easy a way out (and uncomfortably close to euthanasia). The hospice advocate David Dempsey,[38] for example, has argued that "death with dignity is meaningful only if we know of what dignity consists in a terminal life.... The good death is not necessarily an easy death; it is one which permits a person to die in character.... At what point should the leukemia patient be allowed to die naturally; that is, in pain? When does life cease to have quality and meaning? Sudden death does not answer these questions." In addition, hospice care rests on a significant amount of residual work performed by supportive relatives and large volunteer pools (mostly women). Hospice is also for patients who are dying but not for those who want to hasten the dying process. From its inception, hospice care has steered away from the right-to-die movement. For example, the sociologist Anne Munley describes the emotional problems of a 78-year-old patient with prostate cancer: "Patient wants to die now; says to nurses, 'Why can't it be now?' Depressed, sometimes refuses medications."[39] The interdisciplinary team decided during a hospice-care meeting that the solution for this patient was to initiate relaxation therapy and arrange for a psychiatric consultation, presumably to treat the death wish.

Different hospice programs are now integrated into the general health-care landscape. A major issue during the early years of hospice was financing. When researchers showed that, overall, hospice care is less expensive than traditional care (although in individual cases the care might become more expensive),[40] Medicare and private insurers instituted reimbursement structures for hospice services. The services covered, ironically, are mainly physical care, not the social-psychological caregiving related to grieving and bereavement. Thus, "as hospice programs became popular and became integrated with the health care system, those aspects of hospice services that were not consistent with traditional health care values were downplayed or ignored."[41] Instead of an alternative to traditional hospital care, hospice is now at best a supplement to hospital care and often emulates the problems of the past (for example, by focusing on "curing" the pains of dying). Also important is that sudden death remains unaddressed by hospice advocates; nor has sudden death been the focus of the next mobilization around death awareness.

RIGHT-TO-DIE MOVEMENT

In the nineties, a new wave of death awareness engulfed the United States. Although alienation from death was still a general sentiment, the solution became withdrawing or withholding life support or actively assisting in death. The first decades of experience with hospice care demonstrated that the hospice movement filled a void but still had limitations: hospice care often came too late, was out of reach for the under- or uninsured, and remained anathema to core medical values.[42] Of the two million people who die yearly in the United States, the most optimistic figures suggest that hospice programs collectively serve only about 200,000 patients annually.[43] Throughout the seventies and eighties, the practice of secretively—or not so secretively—aiding persons with degenerative or terminal illnesses to die gained public attention as several spokespeople brought these practices, and the laws forbidding them, into the open.

The National Hemlock Society is the best-known organization advocating a do-it-yourself approach to death. Started in 1980 by the journalist Derek Humphry, the society was the outgrowth of Humphry's experience in helping his cancer-afflicted first wife take her life, a story he tells in *Jean's Way*,[44] a book about her suicide. The organization's goal originally was to inform terminally ill people about taking their own lives. To that end, Humphry published *Final Exit*,[45] which became a

best-seller when it was reissued in 1991. The book details the practical-
ities of securing enough sleeping pills and the need for a back-up plan
with a plastic bag. Today, the organization lobbies to legalize physician-
assisted suicide.

The most vocal spokesperson for the recent resurgence of the right-
to-die movement is the retired pathologist Dr. Jack Kevorkian, who
first drew public attention when he assisted Janet Adkins's suicide in
1990 with the aid of his suicide machine in the back of his old Volks-
wagen van.[46] Adkins's was living with the early stages of Alzheimer's
disease. She had sought pharmacological treatment, which had failed,
and after a single conversation, Kevorkian agreed to help her to die.
The suicide apparatus first delivered an intravenous infusion of saline
solution. An anesthetic (thiopental) was ready to flow when Adkins
pushed the button; the potassium chloride, which caused a lethal heart-
rhythm disorder, automatically followed one minute later. Later ver-
sions of the suicide machine relied on carbon monoxide. Since then,
Kevorkian has assisted in a growing number of people's deaths. After
several acquittals for assisted suicide, Kevorkian was finally convicted
in 1999 after he terminated a patient's life with an injection on a television show.

In contrast to the ethically suspect and media-savvy positions of
Humphrey and Kevorkian, Dr. Timothy E. Quill, a former hospice physician in Rochester, New York, has taken a more thoughtful and compassionate position in the debate on physician-assisted suicide. Quill entered the spotlight in 1991 with his account of counseling and providing
lethal drugs for "Diane," which was published in the *New England Journal of Medicine.* [47] Diane had been Quill's patient for eight years when
she was diagnosed with leukemia. She rejected the chemotherapy which
offered a projected long-term survival rate of 25 percent, and instead
opted for hospice care. Diane feared losing control in a lingering-death
trajectory, and when she brought up suicide with Quill, he suggested
she contact the National Hemlock Society. The next week, Diane called
Quill with a request for barbiturates to sleep, which the doctor recognized as an essential ingredient in a Hemlock Society suicide. Over the
following weeks, Quill repeatedly asked Diane whether she was indeed
making an informed decision and made sure that she knew the exact
dosage needed for suicide. The last months of Diane's life were spent
with friends and family: her son stayed home from college, and her
husband worked at home so that they could spend time together. Even-

tually, Diane died after taking the barbiturates that Quill had provided to her and after sending her husband and son out for a walk. In this and other case studies,[48] Quill argues that assisting patients to die should never take the place of extensive comfort and hospice care, but that if a patient demands a lethal dose, a physician should provide it. The physician's goals are to help the patient remain comfortable and in control and to allow death with as much dignity as possible.

Recognizing that access to medical care is currently too inequitable and that many doctor-patient relationships are too impersonal for legalized active euthanasia, Quill and his colleagues have argued for a more widespread acceptance of physician-assisted suicide. Their program rests on a case-based approach within the confines of informed decision making. Other advocates of assisted suicide envision a health-care system in which assisted suicide is one more health-care choice available for patients. Although Washington and California have defeated initiatives to legalize assisted suicide, Oregon voters approved a Death with Dignity Act in 1994 and left it in place during a 1997 referendum.[49]

As the right-to-die movement gained momentum, an important chorus of dissent came from disability advocates. The disability-rights movement has been very critical of the presumed "right" to die if this right is not counterbalanced with a "right" to life for the disabled and the elderly. Nancy Mairs points out that "if, after consulting with family, spiritual counselors, and medical personnel, a diabetic with gangrenous legs may ask for an easeful death, he should also be fully supported in his decision to live as an amputee, confident that he can continue to work, shop, attend church, take his wife out for dinner and a movie, just as he has always done. Only in a society that respects, and enables, these choices are atrocities against the disabled truly unthinkable."[50]

While most of the media in recent years has focused on different kinds of assisted suicide, the more passive variation of withdrawing and withholding life supports has received legal support with the Patient Self-Determination Act (PSDA). This act is a federal law affecting all health-care agencies that receive any federal (Medicare, Medicaid, or other) funding. As an outgrowth of the Nancy Cruzan case,[51] the federal government now mandates that health-care providers inform patients about their right to refuse and accept treatment, even when they have lost decision-making capacity. The goal of the PSDA is to motivate people to make their wishes about treatment known in advance, but not to force them to do so. This information needs to be given when patients first enroll in pre-paid HMOs; when they receive care from hospices or hospitals; and before they receive care from home-health agencies or nursing homes. In addition, the PSDA mandates that care providers document in the medical records whether or not an advance directive has been executed, and that they maintain written policies and procedures to implement patients' rights to accept or refuse treatment and to make advance directives. The law does not apply to individual physicians' practices. The PSDA makes it more difficult to ignore a patient's values and preferences and stimulates thought and discussion about what care is acceptable. This law strengthens a number of burgeoning informal initiatives, such as physicians' "do not resuscitate" (DNR) orders written in patient files, which are aimed at reducing indiscriminate resuscitative efforts.

The PSDA has been criticized because the timing of informing patients is bad: the stress of hospital admission is the worst possible time.[52] Typically, an unskilled employee is asked to administer an extra form and has no incentive to engage in a philosophical discussion about end-of-life care. In addition, the federal government does not provide any penalties for not honoring advance directives. Care providers are penalized only if they do not inform people about advance directives. In addition, Congress did not allocate money for a federal educational campaign. Finally, in medical practice, advance directives are often too vague and difficult to interpret, or they are kept in a place where they cannot be accessed. Although these documents were formulated to prevent the overuse of CPR in hospitals, I will show in Chapter 5 that advance directives have failed to reduce resuscitative care.

The second wave of death awareness is still making headlines. Researchers have found that Kevorkian now personifies death,[53] while death autonomy has become a cause that attracts ballot initiatives. Although hospice and right-to-die advocates are often philosophically and politically in opposite camps, activists on both sides agree about which deaths need to be avoided. These agreements about "good" deaths form the basis for the exclusion of sudden death from their campaigns.

THE "GOOD" DEATH

In the embracing of the hospice and right-to-die model, certain aspects of the dying experience—abandonment, lack of communication, pain management, and suffering—have been deemed more problematic than others. The result is a remarkable consensus among social scientists, medical communities, and the general public with respect to the social problem of contemporary dying. The main problematic issue in death and dying is still the abandonment of people in hospitals when their condition turns terminal. When Kübler-Ross was hospitalized in the mid-nineties for a severe stroke, she experienced firsthand how dying patients were still ignored and, ironically, psychologically redefined:

> After teaching doctors and nurses for decades, I was in the hospital after my stroke, and it was like my work was non-existent. The nurses never came to see their patients. They would just sit out there in front of their computers. I had this frozen arm and incredible pain. If you blew on my left arm, I would scream. The nurse told me I was holding my hand in a funny way—which is typical of stroke patients—and she sat on my arm! I slugged her with my good arm and yelled, 'That hurts like hell!' She said, 'Oh, you're becoming combative,' and brought in two fat nurses who tried to sit on it again. If I had a pistol, I would have shot them. When I left the hospital, I was so depressed. It was like my work for four decades had gone down the drain. Nobody learned anything.[54]

She admitted that her own experience made her appreciate "anger" more than "acceptance."

Hospitals, with their intensive-care units, are construed as the symbolic epicenters of "unnatural" places to die. They have become breeding grounds for ethical dilemmas in life-and-death decision making and the allocation of scarce medical resources. As Renée Anspach shows in her ethnography of life-and-death decision making in neonatal intensive-care units, the staff elicits parents' assent to decisions that have already been made. Anspach concludes, "In many ways, neonatal intensive care epitomizes the kinds of dilemmas that arise in the high technology medical settings that have come to proliferate in our times. A culture that rewards science, technology, teaching, and learning, and that devalues interaction with patients, is coupled with a social structure that places barriers between physicians, patients, and parents. While some decisions are relatively unproblematic, all too often outcomes ensue that adversely affect the lives of all concerned."[55] In general, the hospital's organization, with its rigid visiting hours and its prohibitions against overnight stays for visitors, further alienates relatives from participating in the last moments with the dying person.

Over the past decades, technology has been singled out as the main villain in narratives about contemporary death and dying. Medical technology is overwhelmingly considered alienating, objectifying, fragmenting, and above all "unnatural." The sociologist David Wendell Moller is the most fervent believer in the power of technology to ruin the dying experience: "Clearly, technology is the driving force in medical education. Clearly, technological activism is the dominant factor which shapes the world view of physicians. Clearly, the technological orientation of the medical profession is the major force which shapes physician interaction with dying patients. Thus, despite the realities of normlessness and the appearance of differences in the approach of doctors to the treatment of the dying patient, technology is the pre-eminent tool used in the management of the terminally ill."[56] Moller labels this "technological force" "the save-at-all costs orientation" that leads to "aggressive," "dehumanizing," and "depersonalized" treatment.[57] Others "clearly" agree with Moller. They explain that "technological death"[58] facilitates "the loss of the dignity of the individual,"[59] "loss of self possession and conscious integrity,"[60] "depersonalization,"[61] "psychological mutilation and scars for unprepared family members,"[62] and "avoidance and distancing"[63] and ultimately turns health-care workers into "technocrats"[64] or "plumbers making repairs, connecting tubes and flushing out clogged systems, with no questions asked."[65] Basically, "it is beyond the power of technology to solve the essentially moral problems of the dying—problems of sentiment, of conscience, and of convictions about what is right. Technology cannot substitute for love, tenderness, and compassion."[66]

Technology and, to a lesser extent, the hospital institution have been singled out as the sources of distortion for our experience of death and dying. But in contrast with the past, which fed off a general uneasy feeling of alienation, hundreds of thousands of copies of Kübler-Ross's works, several thousand hospices, and the activities of Dr. "Death" Kevorkian[67] have helped promote a specific idea of a "good"—or, at least, a "better"—death. Susan Sontag pointed out that lingering death trajectories became the dominant cultural metaphor for dying.[68] The thanatologist (somebody who studies death) Avery D. Weisman introduced the notion of an "appropriate" death.[69] He believed that most people would choose for themselves a death that includes several facets: it would be relatively pain-free, suffering would be reduced, and emotional and social impoverishment would be kept at a minimum. The ethicist Daniel Callahan lists the following criteria for his ideal form of death, the "peaceful" death: it is meaningful to the dying person, the person is treated with respect and dignity, the person is conscious until very near the time of death, the death matters to others, the dying person is surrounded by friends and relatives without being an undue burden on them, the death occurs quickly and is not drawn out, the pain is bearable, and, finally, the dying process occurs in a society that does not "dread death and that provides support in its rituals and public practices for comforting the dying, and, after death, their friends and families."[70] The sociologist Allan Kellehaer constructed his own list of five characteristics of the ideal–typical good death: awareness of dying, personal preparations and social adjustments, financial and legal preparations, closure on employment and other responsibilities, and making formal and informal farewells.[71] Those academic models reflect among the wider public. Robert Kastenbaum and C. Normand[72] surveyed students enrolled in death-education courses about how they depicted their own deaths. Like Callahan, the typical respondent "expected to die in old age, at home, quickly, with the companionship of loved ones, while remaining alert, and not experiencing pain or any other symptoms."

While these contemporary notions have idealized forms of dying as "good" deaths and have promoted the hospice and assisted suicide as solutions for the problems of contemporary dying, they exclude entire sets of dying experiences that do not fit the prevalent definition of the problems. As Michael Bury observed, "The greatest danger lies in the fact that the Good Death, far from extending the remit of professional power, may act as an ideological gloss, covering the distress and agony that people continue to face with or without formal care."[73] Sudden deaths in particular have become invisible to a thanatological treatment blinded by the flashlight of hospice care and the right to die. For some thanatologists, sudden death is unproblematic because, in its "pure" form, a quick and unexpected passing comes close to the culturally prevalent image of the "good" death. Sudden death is swift and relatively painless. The dying person does not have the opportunity to contemplate the possibility of death. The dying leave life in the middle of activity, not at the end of a debilitating, lingering trajectory. Therefore, nothing need be done—no acceptance, no autonomy. Even if we could find a problem, the practical barriers to instituting a hospice or right-to-die program for those who die suddenly seem insurmountable. How can one organize the preparatory death work required to address the spiritual and social needs of the people dying a sudden death when sudden death occurs unexpectedly? How can one increase patient autonomy when the patient is unconscious?

Sudden death might once have been "good" in its ideal form, but over the past decades, sudden death has become increasingly medicalized through an increased reliance on resuscitative efforts. This medicalization now reflects the problems that plagued the lingering dying trajectories to the extent that sudden deaths are now also prime examples of deaths to avoid. Whenever somebody falls over, anyone who knows CPR is expected to check for an open airway, breathing, and a pulse. When those vital signs are missing, CPR is to begin, with the emergency medical system alerted. A resuscitative effort continues with drug therapies, defibrillators, and intravenous pumps while paramedics or emergency technicians transport the patient to an emergency department. While the patient is the focus of a reviving attempt, relatives and friends are kept separate in a counseling or family room. Only when the patient has died (or in rare cases has been stabilized) are these significant others ushered into the resuscitation room to pay their last respects or visit. The patient who is declared dead at the end of a resuscitative effort, has died among health-care providers. A resuscitative effort following a sudden collapse thus has all the properties of a feared technological death with abandonment in the hospital.

In sum, sudden death does not fit in the current death-awareness discourse. In its pure form, it is very close to our contemporary conception of a "good" death, while in its current practice it is the exemplar of the death to be avoided. The consequence is that we now have two parallel, opposite universes of dying: lingering and sudden death. Death at the end of a lingering trajectory is part of a battle about where and how to die. Its three main alternatives are: the hospital death, the hospice death, and the assisted or self-induced suicide death. Sudden death, in contrast, provides no comparable options. This way of passing has never erupted into debate because it falls outside the confines of the death-awareness agenda. Instead, sudden death is overwhelmingly medicalized, and saving lives has become the ideal. Yet the lack of attention by the death-awareness movement has exacerbated the problems with resuscitation. As I will show in the next chapters, the emergency medical profession has had free rein to define sudden death.

Toward a Dignified Sudden Death?

Sudden death is now solidly under medical jurisdiction, but what if we open a dialogue between resuscitative efforts and death awareness?

How can sudden death become more meaningful? How can we keep the valuable aspects of the death-awareness movement and add sudden death to that agenda? If our goal is to make all death—including sudden death—a more dignified and compassionate passing, we will need to change some of the assumptions that underpin the current death-awareness movement. Specifically, we will need to revise our opinions about the "goodness" of certain kinds of dying.

This task is easier than it seems because the anti-technology/anti-hospital position of the death-awareness movement clashes with the reality of hospice care and assisted suicide. The "natural" pre–Victorian deathbed scene made sense in small communities tied together by strong religious traditions. In contemporary secularized societies, however, we cannot transplant such death communities and still expect the medical care we have taken for granted during the past century. Not only are hospices modeled after hospitals, but hospice care and the right-to-die movement also depend on technology and advanced medical care. "Good" deaths now require a relatively painless expiring. The management of pain, however, depends on more aggressive pharmacological intervention than the standard of care in traditional pre-hospice medicine. Indeed, palliative-care physicians are often now pain specialists and have helped launch pain management as a medical subdiscipline. A similar critique can be made about the assisted-death movement. Kevorkian hides behind a suicide machine while the do-it-yourself Hemlock Society depends on physicians to prescribe the barbiturates necessary for a painless death. Both Kevorkian and Quill prefer that a physician assist the dying. These alternative kinds of dying represent a refocus instead of abandonment of technology and professional medical care.

If we want to add resuscitative care to the death-awareness agenda, the first task is not to fall for the pitfalls of a naive technological determinism in which technology is intrinsically evil and distorts the current dying experience. Nor do we want to glorify technology as the savior for dignified dying. Our goal is to examine the different ways in which technology transforms the dying experience and to foster those aspects that would create a more dignified and compassionate event. *A dignified and compassionate sudden death implies that the possibility of death is made explicit, treatment choices are reached with all parties involved, the dying person's wishes are honored, and relatives and friends are included in the last moments, if not as care-providers, then at least as witnesses.* Like Glaser and Strauss, Sudnow, Kübler-Ross, and others before us, we need to enter

EDs and examine resuscitative interventions that rarely succeed in saving lives. We need to look at what it means to die a medicalized sudden death. We need to measure the margin of change in these life-and-death encounters. But first we need to understand the origin of the belief that death is reversible. As I will show in the next two chapters, enrolling entire societies in the belief that every sudden death is a premature death and conditioning people to massage chests and put their mouths on the mouths of strangers was one of Western medicine's major achievements in the late twentieth century. Universal CPR was indeed an accomplishment of medical power, especially because, in reality, lives are rarely saved.

2 The Search for the Best Resuscitation Technique

MEDICAL TEXTS regularly locate the origins of the current resuscitation techniques in biblical passages such as this one about the Prophet Elisha:[1]

> 32 And when E-li-sha was come into the house, behold, the child was dead, and laid upon his bed.
> 33 He went in therefore, and shut the door upon them twain, and prayed unto the Lord.
> 34 And he went up, and lay upon the child, and put his mouth upon his mouth, and his eyes upon his eyes, and his hands upon his hands: and he stretched himself upon the child; and the flesh of the child waxed warm.
> 35 Then he returned, and walked in the house to and fro; and went up, and stretched himself upon him: and the child opened his eyes.[2]

Although this biblical passage shows a vague similarity to current resuscitation techniques, locating the roots of reviving in the Hebrew Bible provides a false sense of historical continuity and misrepresents the role of religion in the resuscitation project. The current reliance on mouth-to-mouth ventilation stems from the late fifties rather than from ancient times. For long periods of history, mouth-to-mouth ventilation was vehemently opposed and actually forbidden. Thus, instead of a simple linear history, resuscitation techniques have followed a messier path. What people not so long ago considered to be the most scientific resuscitation technique is now dismissed as ineffective and even dangerous. And what others in earlier times disregarded as insignificant and misguided is now embraced as the best way to revive people. Ironically, religious beliefs rendered resuscitation a non-issue for centuries. Most ancient religions, including the Judeo-Christian tradition, considered it blasphemous to alter the boundary between life and death. The power over death distinguished the mortals from the gods. The severest punishments were often reserved for those who had violated the boundaries of life. Not until the scientific revolution in the late eighteenth century did resuscitation become a possibility. Thus, early Christians most likely viewed Elisha's actions, such as his revival of the son of Zarapath's widow in 1 Kings 17:17-22, as instances of divine power, not as an example to be emulated by human beings. In ancient Israel, disease, healing, and resurrection were Yahweh's exclusive responsibility.

Significant, however, is that contemporary medical researchers chose to locate the origins of resuscitation in the Bible. Resuscitating aims to alter by human means what for most of history has been considered an unchangeable divine prerogative. In this context, a biblical story is strategically useful as a rhetorical charm for those who dare to trespass the boundary between life and death. Resuscitation has never been an obvious choice and even now is marred by ethical controversies. To engage in resuscitative efforts implies that human beings put faith in technical and pharmacological interventions to overcome death. Death, instead of a final and irrevocable passage, becomes a process manipulable by humans. Resuscitation implies the recognition of a distinction between the moment when the signs of death set in (clinical death) and irreversible death of the human organism (biological death). How did people in Western societies move from believing that death was untouchable and predetermined to making resuscitative care a common procedure in emergency medicine?

The historical breakthrough that made resuscitation a viable project occurred in the late eighteenth century, when the first organizations centralized lifesaving at a community level. These societies—organized to educate the population and promote local efforts—are important for two reasons. First, with the new organizations, isolated resuscitative practices[3] gained visibility and required the approval of religious authorities. Civil authorities also needed to be convinced that resuscitating was a harmless activity and not a license for murder. Founders of the new lifesaving organizations were able to persuade their detractors that saving lives that would otherwise be lost did not violate church dogma but was a noble, philanthropic activity. At the end of the eighteenth century, physicians promoted the belief that human intervention in the area between life and death was appropriate and possible. Second, these organizations centralized and explicitly encouraged the search for new and better resuscitation technology. They started with the conviction that under certain circumstances death did not need to be final, and then analyzed available practices with laboratory support. Resuscitation techniques prospered in the dialogue between technology and a growing belief that death is reversible.

The moment of truth for resuscitation occurred at lake- and river-fronts where lives were saved through approved interventions. Resuscitating would have remained a pointless project if its advocates had not been able to reverse the dying process and save human lives. Every successful resuscitative effort became, literally, living proof of technology's promise and fueled the search for better techniques. But was every failed resuscitative effort proof of its failure? Not exactly. The cultural turn toward resuscitation techniques and the search for the best life-saving technology marks the historical origins of a discrepancy between attempted resuscitation and the relatively few lives it saves. Rather than chart an instance of linear technological progress, the historical succession of resuscitation methods illustrates the management of successes and failures. The accomplishment of the resuscitation project was to turn lifesaving into a taken-for-granted activity, to make resuscitation a morally sanctioned routine.

THE ROYAL HUMANE SOCIETY

A wreck has happened—by some mismanagement, a sudden squall, a boat has upset the joyous party—look at the frightful scene, hear their loud shrieks for help! See the convulsed grasps of each! With uplifted hands to Heaven, vehemently they cry for mercy! The piercing tones of one among them are distinctly heard and known—they are the moans of a beloved child—the parents drop on the beach with deathlike torpor:—the feelings of the spectators are harrowed up, dismay is in every countenance!

No boat can venture forth. A point of time—another wave decides their fate! At this impending moment a life-boat is providentially obtained: instantly it is put in readiness, and dares to face the hurricane—the sinking limbs are rescued—and the living bodies conveyed to receive, through the instructions and other aids of the Humane Society, that peculiar reparation, which so dreadful an attack on the delicate organization of life had made essential.[4]

Because of their proximity to oceans, lakes, ponds, brooks, and ubiquitous canals, the Netherlands and Britain always have had many drowning accidents. In 1767, the Dutch founded a society in Amsterdam for resuscitating the drowned.[5] Within four years, the Dutch organization had claimed that 150 people had been saved by its recommendations. The victims had been immersed in water from fifteen minutes to an hour and a half. A British counterpart—the Society for the Recovery of Persons Apparently Drowned, renamed the Royal Humane Society for the Apparently Dead—followed in 1774.[6] These societies were the first organized attempts at centralizing resuscitation knowledge, and the British society played a major role in the development of resuscitation techniques until the Second World War.

In 1774, the founder and driving force behind the British society, the London apothecary Dr. William Hawes, reminded his fellow society members that in the previous year 125 people had drowned in the London area: "suppose but one in ten restored, what man would think the designs of this society unimportant, were himself, his relation or his friend—that one?"[7] In the late eighteenth century, however, this powerful personalized argument was insufficient to garner wide support for the Royal Humane Society. Instead, Hawes and his fellow society members faced strong resistance. When Hawes died in 1808, the society members recalled, "Our first object and chief difficulty were to remove that destructive incredulity which prevailed. Our attempts were treated, not only by the *vulgar*, but by some of *the learned*, even by *men of eminence* as physicians and philosophers, as idle and visionary, and placed upon a level with professing to raise the dead. The well-authenticated narratives from abroad were considered as confabulous; or, at least, as greatly exaggerated. Such prejudices were first to be removed; and they could only be removed by uncontestible facts of our own."[8]

Faced with a skeptical response, Hawes and his colleagues needed to convince themselves and others that lives could be saved through human intervention. Demonstration thus became the hallmark of the nascent society.[9] Because of the initial derision and ridicule, they offered money to persuade people to report drownings, to pull victims out of the water and attempt to revive them. The treasurer of the Royal Humane Society also received letters with testimonies of children, men, and women who had slipped into water, fallen through ice, or were found floating in rivers, lakes, and seas. Other stories dealt with suicides, hangings, poisonings, and victims of lightning and suffocation. For example:

Dear Sir,   Fakenham, April 14th 1802

On the 12th of April, a storm of hail suddenly came on, succeeded by a most vivid flash of lightning.—In about five minutes I was requested to visit J. Mitchell, who was then struck dead with lightning; and had been an apparent corpse half an hour. A dead cold pervaded the body, the pupils of his eyes were much dilated, the countenance exhibiting ghastly appearance.

Visible marks of the electric fluid were on his knee angles, and feet, resembling those following the explosion of gunpowder. I commenced with ardour the Resuscitative Plans recommended by the R.H.S. which, by assiduous perseverance for three quarters of an hour, was productive of returning animation, convulsions, interrupted respiration, diffusion of heat, and languid circulation.—My restored patient was confined to his bed some days; but by medical attention his life and health were perfectly restored.[10]

For unsuccessful outcomes, some of the narratives detailed autopsy information. These stories were verified in a different letter by learned men (a priest, physician, or army officer) or by three credible witnesses. For the Royal Humane Society, the bundle of testimonies and the tally of successful interventions and failures became proof that lives could indeed be saved through human intervention.

Despite such proof, the question of whether human intervention was appropriate remained unanswered. At issue was not an ethical objection to interference in the end of life but a religious concern about God's will. Church critics considered the claim of restoring life blasphemous because only the Creator could give or take life. Hawes countered with an argument about suspended animation. He and his successors sharply distinguished resuscitating from reanimating and reviving from resurrection: "The former is merely to re-kindle the flame of a taper, by gently fanning the ignited wick; the latter to re-animate a corpse, after the vital spark is totally extinct."[11] The former belonged to the domain of the physician or any other trained person; the latter was God's province. In their publications, society members emphasized restoring *temporarily suspended* life of the *apparently* dead. Igniting the wick of life became the motto of the society, and on its medals the society printed "Lateat Scintillula Florsan" (Possibly a Little Spark Might Yet Lie Hid). Resuscitation techniques were effective only when the person was not yet totally dead, a condition that implied that not everyone could be revived.

The Royal Humane Society further secured the church's support with a blessing of the society's initiatives during an annual church service. But in 1803, when Dr. R. Strive gave the sermon to praise the Royal Humane Society, he became the subject of a religious critique[12] because he located the practice of the rescue in biblical events such as the revival of the Shunnamite child by Elisha. Critics immediately contested the comparison because the biblical tale was considered a miracle and thus had nothing to do with the work of the Royal Humane Society. Dr. Strive recanted and clarified the issue in an appendix to the sermon.[13] The society members also dismissed miraculous rescues, such as revival after being immersed in water for more than two hours, as reported by Shakespeare:

> Death May Usurp on Nature many Hours
> And yet the Fire of Life Kindle Again.
> The Overpressed Spirits. I have heard
> Of an Egyptian had Nine Hours been Dead,
> By good Appliance was Recovered.[14]

An early society member, the Quaker physician Antony Fothergill, diversified the arguments for resuscitating by pointing to examples in nature, which provided simple means of restoring life for frozen eels, which could be brought to life by slow warming. Rescuers simply seized on those practices and redefined them as an art: the art of resuscitating. Fothergill reasoned that if God had bestowed simple animals with the ability to revive, humans could safely engage in resuscitative efforts as well.

Attempting to revive people was then not blasphemous but a noble, morally approved human practice. Like feeding the hungry and clothing the naked, reviving temporarily dead people became defined as a Christian charity, a religiously sound activity. The church eventually not only tolerated but also praised the work of the Royal Humane Society, especially its efforts to interrupt and revive potential suicides. According to the Church of England, a successful rescue meant not only that a human being was "reconciled to life and public utility" but also that a soul was saved. By 1809, the members of the Royal Humane Society would give the suicidal person a Bible and summon a priest when encountering a suicide attempt.

Hawes appealed to government officials with a different set of arguments: he pointed out that it was their responsibility to preserve the lives of their constituents. When the objection was raised that resuscitative aid would be a good alibi for a murderer, Hawes countered that the organization's guidelines would allow rescuers to save otherwise dead murder victims and thus facilitate police work. Hawes also played on fears of live burial. He warned the general public not to assume that death had occurred before "putrefaction" had set in. Especially in cases of fainting, convulsions, "fevers arising in weak habits," smallpox, and even old age, people might accidentally be buried alive. Several countries passed legislation requiring that burial be delayed up to three days after death. In the eyes of government officials, the Royal Humane Society became an important philanthropic society aimed at preserving the public good, and in 1787 King George III lent the society his patronage. Through its efforts, workers and even dignitaries could be saved, and the establishment of similar rescue societies in other countries, including America,[15] added glory to the British empire. The society also capitalized on every opportunity for favorable notice. In 1806, it awarded its gold medal to Alexander I, czar of Russia, who allegedly had risked his life to save a Polish peasant from drowning.[16] The czar received the medal in 1814 on a visit to London. Early society members also invited distinguished persons to become honorary members.

In its crucial first years, the Royal Humane Society reported impressive survival rates. Between 1774 and 1793, the rescue organization gathered 1,706 cases, and 747, or 43.7 percent, were considered successful reviving attempts.[17] To put those successes in perspective, we need to keep in mind that the concept of a resuscitative effort was very broad in the eighteenth century. Resuscitating did not only imply a situation in which life was suspended by cardiac arrest but also included people thrown into the water during a storm, screaming to be rescued, and people who had lost consciousness because of smoke inhalation. These events qualified as resuscitative efforts because if the rescuer had not intervened, the victim would likely have died.[18] While adopting a broad definition of resuscitation, early members of the humane societies recognized that not every person could be saved. The techniques seemed to be most efficient at the waterfront. Thus, while the term "resuscitation" covered a wide category of rescue situations, the effort was also more specifically associated with drownings.

The credibility of the early rescuers rested on the successful application of recommended techniques. Increasing the survival rate became the motivation behind the continuous search for the best resuscitation method, because with every life saved, the platform of the Royal Humane Society would be revalidated. The society thus had a quest for the "best" resuscitation technique, but just what was it? Clearly, the technique that saved the most lives was the best, but in practice, criteria used to determine a technique's effectiveness were related only partly to the success of a technique in saving human lives, either in the laboratory or in the field. The success of a technique was not always discriminatory, because all innovators promised that each new method would save more lives than the current practice. A simple comparison of successes between new and old techniques was virtually impossible because comparative data were nonexistent or, when available, were not interpreted.

In addition, techniques had different scopes, used novel principles, and thus applied different definitions to resuscitation. If experimental data and clinical statistics could not explain the use of one resuscitation method over another, what factors were decisive in establishing clinical standards? In some instances, decisive factors seem to be a combination of deductive reasoning and social–political clout. In other cases, educational, moral, or aesthetic considerations gave one technique the edge over the other.

These non-performance factors widened the gap between justifying resuscitative efforts in the laboratory and practicing resuscitation in the field. Over time, just the promise that a new technique would result in more saved lives became sufficient. Whether lives were actually saved, and at what cost, were not relevant questions. The promise that more lives could be saved with technical innovation seduced many into adapting new techniques and revising previous recommendations when alternatives appeared on the scene. The result was to broaden the scope of resuscitation and make ever greater claims for new techniques. Gradually, the qualifiers (only some lives could be saved under certain conditions) disappeared.

THE RESUSCITATION TECHNIQUES OF THE ROYAL HUMANE SOCIETY

The Vital Principle

In its first report, the Royal Humane Society recommended the Dutch methods for resuscitation: warmth, artificial ventilation, administering tobacco smoke rectally or fumigating it,[19] rolling the body over a barrel, rubbing the body, and bleeding from a vein, along with the accessory means of vomiting, sneezing, and administering internal stimulants. In addition, the Royal Humane Society also explicitly forbade the use of other methods such as inversion or suspending the body from the heels;[20] waving ammonia under the nose; and tickling the patient's throat with a feather. Although the Royal Humane Society lacked enforcement power, it published warnings about the harms of using the wrong techniques. In light of the search for the best means to resuscitate, it is noteworthy that all of the initially recommended methods, with the exception of warmth and rubbing, would eventually make the list of forbidden practices. Used nevertheless, a reviewer observed that "not one of these cases where forbidden methods were applied resulted in failure."[21]

In the eighteenth century, warming the body seemed the key to survival. Keeping the body warm aligned with the Greek physician Galen's still widely known theory that body warmth is the necessary characteristic of vitality. For the next century, society members debated whether the complement to warming the body was artificial ventilation or some other method. Besides a cooling body, the loss of breathing seemed the most discernible sign of death, but its importance in a successful resuscitation remained ambiguous. Referring to nature, Fothergill made a strong claim for stimulating respiration not just with natural air but with "dephlogisticated" air (oxygen): "The vital breeze which nature pours to save, the breathless victim from th' untimely grave."[22] Apparently, however, Fothergill did not believe that artificial respiration was sufficient to restore life because he presented a plan requiring a team of seven people executing fifteen steps to revive a patient.[23] Next to warming the body, artificial respiration with bellows (or preferably with a special dephlogisticated air machine) was the preferred method if the rescuer was alone. If more people were available, two of them should use an "electrical machine" over the heart to restore the cardiac functions.[24]

Over the next century, the society advocated a series of contradictory recommendations about stimulating respiratory function. Initially, artificial ventilation was mouth-to-mouth ventilation:

> The subject being placed in one of other of these advantageous circumstances as speedily as possible, various stimulating methods should next be employed. The most effacious are—to blow with force into the lungs, by applying the mouth to that part of the patient, closing his nostrils with one hand, and gently expelling the air again by pressing the chest with the other, imitating the strong breathing of the healthy person: the medium of a handkerchief or cloth may be used to render the operation less indelicate.[25]

The mouth-to-mouth method, however, soon lost favor. According to early reports, until the founding of the Royal Humane Society, mouth-to-mouth ventilation was rarely used to revitalize drowning victims and was instead associated with removing mucus from the airways of stillborn babies. The first accounts probably came from Paracelsus in 1530[26] and Vesalius in 1543, who inflated the lungs of animals by blowing intermittently into a tube in the trachea.[27] In 1744, Fothergill noted how Dr. Tossach of Alloa had used mouth-to-mouth ventilation to revive a miner who was apparently dead from suffocation. Fothergill also mentioned the use of bellows as an alternative means for artificial ventilation but preferred mouth-to-mouth ventilation. Bellows had long been known to anatomists as instruments for keeping animals alive during experiments.

Soon after the establishment of the Royal Humane Society, in 1776, Dr. John Hunter and Dr. W. Cullen from Edinburgh both recommended the bellows as more effective than mouth-to-mouth ventilation. By 1812, mouth-to-mouth ventilation was totally out of favor because the exhaled breath was considered poisonous. The bellows method, in turn, fell into disfavor in 1837 after several French researchers determined that an animal could be killed by suddenly inflating its lungs and that the effort could produce emphysema and pneumothorax in dead animals. Artificial respiration in general was further discredited when the influential president of the Royal Humane Society, Sir Benjamin Brodie, stated that ventilation itself could not restart a stopped heart. He believed that the heart stopped two to three minutes after respiration ceased, at which point artificial respiration was ineffective. Reviewing the resuscitative attempts from 1830 to 1855, the president of the Royal Humane Society, Dr. Dalrymple, wrote, "It is a singular fact that one of our most active and useful medical assistants, Mr. Woolley, in all the cases in which he has been successful in restoring suspended animation, has never performed the operation of inflation of the lungs, and in all these cases where he did use the bellows, his exertions were of none avail."[28] In this period, treatment began with immersion in a bath at about 100 degrees Fahrenheit. To the amazement of later researchers, "the results during this period show no increase in the number of unsuccessful cases of resuscitation."[29] Not only did artificial ventilation have little effect, but more victims survived their drowning episodes without it.

In 1857, Dr. Marshall Hall noted the absence of artificial respiration in the rescue organization's recommendations and conducted a series of experiments on corpses that resulted in a new theory of death by drowning. He concluded that drowning was similar to anaesthesia and poisoning because both invoked a discharge of carbon dioxide.[30] He discovered that when the patient was face-up, the tongue and larynx were likely to fall back and occlude the air passage. This response could be avoided when the victim was kept in a face-down position. Hall modified the old practice of "rolling the body" over a barrel into what he called the "postural method." This technique produced expiration by turning the patient in the face-down position and by applying pressure to the back, over the thorax and abdomen. Inspiration commenced the moment the pressure was withdrawn and was completed by rolling the patient on the side. Within a year of his work's publication, Hall was able to attribute twenty-three cases of successful recovery from drowning to his method.

While the society discussed Hall's new method, a young surgeon, Henry S. Silvester, proposed another manual ventilation technique. While dissecting bodies, Silvester developed a method that imitated the natural respiratory movements. Silvester modeled his resuscitation technique on what functioned in life instead of on what failed in death. He selected the face-up posture because he believed that in this position the rescuer could check for airway obstruction. The rescuer stood behind the victim, at the head, grabbed the elbows, and pulled the arms back to the victim's ears to stimulate inspiration. To stimulate expiration, the arms were brought back and pressed upon the chest.[31]

The two competing methods—both supported with sound theories, research results, and an impressive list of successes—posed a new dilemma for the society: which method should it recommend? A committee compared the methods on cadavers and agreed that Silvester's was more effective in ventilating the lungs. The society's analysis further marked a gradual shift from the eighteenth to the nineteenth century. In their deliberations, society members referred to the drowning victims as the "dead" and dropped the word "apparent." They omitted the previous century's reliance on the subtle difference between resuscitating and reanimating, thereby expanding the pool of candidates for resuscitation. Still, Hawes's descendants were well aware that only some victims could be revived because "there is a considerable proportion in which every method fails."[32]

With regard to the problem of whether resuscitating involved only warming the body or should be complemented with artificial respiration, the reviewer of the Royal Humane Society's resuscitation records, Arthur Keith, remained puzzled. He noted in 1909 that every resuscitation technique—forbidden or recommended, physiologically sound or far-fetched, with or without artificial respiration—seemed to be able to save an impressive number of human lives. For example, the Frenchman Laborde introduced tongue traction as a resuscitation method in 1892. The method consisted of "opening the mouth and pulling out the tongue with some degree of force."[33] But because the method could not be explained as beneficial on physiological grounds, the Royal Humane Society put it on the list of forbidden methods. Still, people used the method in France, and Laborde noted success in sixty-three cases. Arthur Keith reflected, "Here, then, is a reputably successful method of resuscitation which its author supports with experimental data and practical application and yet cannot be called a method of artificial respiration."[34]

After a century of debate, the society members agreed that artificial ventilation in addition to warming the body was the best means for reviving drowning victims. The terms "resuscitation" and "artificial respiration" were used interchangeably. For the Royal Humane Society, once the vital principle was settled, the issue became determining which artificial-respiration technique was superior.

The Schafer Technique

When Royal Humane Society members introduced new manual ventilation methods, a succession of committees reviewed the existing techniques and sought to recommend a single best process. The first three committees recommended the Silvester method, justifying their findings with research data and a review of case studies. In 1889, however, Professor Edward A. Schafer[35] oversaw (and eventually became) the fourth review committee. He preferred resuscitation with intermittent pressure exerted on the patient's thorax, with the patient in the face-down position. This method became known as the Schafer prone (face-down)-pressure method.

In several publications, Schafer[36] attempted to refine resuscitation-research methodology. Previously, researchers had used still-warm cadavers or dogs. Schafer instead used volunteers who purposely suppressed the breathing reflex and whose breathing output was measured with displaced tidal air volume.[37] Even with those new research subjects and criteria, however, Schafer's observations seemed inconclusive. The tidal volumes resulting from ten different methods employed on five volunteers obtained a range from 258 ml (mililiter) to 508 ml. The Schafer technique resulted only in the fourth-best results, with an average of 366 ml. Silvester opposed the Schafer method because "[t]he posture of the operator 'athwart the patient,' in respect to the female patient was undesirable."[38] But Schafer brushed off such objections by well-known physicians as "merely pious opinions."[39] Instead, he highlighted measurements he took from a single volunteer showing that his method resulted in the higher tidal volumes—if one used it for five minutes instead of one.[40]

For the first half of the twentieth century, the Schafer prone-pressure method became accepted as the preferred technique for resuscitation in Great Britain, the United States, and other parts of the world.[41] Boy Scout organizations, electric utility workers, firefighters, and other rescue personnel learned to resuscitate with the simple Schafer method.[42] While performing the resuscitative motions, the operator repeated the mantra

Out goes the bad air (compressing the thorax),
in comes the good air (releasing the hands).

After the turn of the century and until the end of the Second World War, only small modifications were made to the Schafer and Silvester techniques. The Schafer method was most popular in Britain, France, Belgium, and the United States, while the Silvester method had supporters in Germany, Holland, and Russia. Thus, at the beginning of the twentieth century, we had a fairly stable set of resuscitation guidelines, with the Schafer method the dominant cultural form. Resuscitations were waterbound and involved manual manipulation of the victim to restore respiration. New methods were developed in the laboratory, later to be presented to rescue organizations for adoption. The criterion for evaluation was the amount of air expelled. Death resulted from a lack of oxygen in the lungs and could easily be measured by, for example, putting a small mirror against the victim's mouth. If the mirror fogged up, the victim was alive and did not need to be resuscitated, only warmed. If the mirror did not fog up, artificial-respiration guidelines needed to be followed.

RESUSCITATION RESEARCH IN THE UNITED STATES

Manual Artificial Ventilation Methods

After the Second World War, research on resuscitation technology shifted from Great Britain to the United States. Between 1940 and 1944, the Council of Physical Medicine gathered case studies from the U.S. Coast Guard and the Chicago, Detroit, and Los Angeles fire departments.[43] In 386 cases, the Schafer technique was used solely or in combination with other methods. Fifty-eight of these cases, or 15 percent, survived. This success rate was rather high. The overall survival rate was 6.7 percent.[44] The council researchers lauded the Schafer method because it allowed the rescuer to start immediately and not to wait until mechanical aids were available. For the same reason, in 1948, the American National Red Cross and the Council on Physical Medicine of the American Medical Association issued a joint statement on resuscitation advising the Red Cross to continue to teach the Schafer method.

Still, the Second World War eroded the popularity of the Schafer method. The war experience had created an especially fruitful climate for a review of existing resuscitation techniques because this war offered many opportunities for accumulating resuscitating experience. For example, many people had drowned as troop ships sank. For centuries, drowning victims had been the most likely to be subject to attempts at resuscitation. Furthermore, the Allies feared that the Germans might use nerve gases capable of paralyzing the respiratory muscles, a problem that artificial ventilation could counteract. Wartime conditions also made it convenient for physicians to produce anesthesia with intravenous barbiturates, products that severely depressed breathing and could lead to sudden death. Again, this effect could be counteracted with an artificial-ventilation technique. Finally, the U.S. Navy and U.S. Army preferred different methods for resuscitation, so military researchers sought to identify the better method. All these factors called for revising existing resuscitation techniques and for decisive clinical evidence of the superiority of one over another.

In 1948, the U.S. Army, together with the National Research Council, organized the first ad hoc conference on resuscitation at which physicians reviewed both manual methods for artificial respiration and mechanical resuscitation devices. Conference participants concluded that they lacked data to choose the best manual technique. Thereafter, four research collaborations, coordinated by Dr. Bruce Dill of Chemical Corps Medical Laboratories, began working on a comparative project.

The researchers divided the existing range of manual methods into two groups. In the first were methods that activated either inspiration or expiration; in the second belonged methods in which the rescuer manipulated both inspiration and expiration. All researchers agreed that the second group produced better results. Archer Gordon's research circle at the University of Illinois discovered that the Schafer method was insufficient to move the dead air in the trachea, so that no fresh oxygenated air entered the lungs. This was an amazing finding. The Schafer technique, which for fifty years had been the dominant resuscitation method and had apparently saved thousands of lives in the United States and abroad, seemed worthless on experimental grounds.[45]

Other findings were less definitive. Differences in the circulatory output did not cause the researchers to recommend one manual artificial-ventilation method over the other. All research collaborations condemned the Silvester method because the patient was kept in a face-up position, which was assumed to cause airway occlusion.[46] Researchers recommended the back-pressure arm-lift but suggested that other resuscitation methods be learned, as no method was effective in all circumstances.

Although the abandonment of the Schafer method constituted a significant change, the first American venture in resuscitation research fit the tradition of the Royal Humane Society. The criteria for a good resuscitative technique, the definition of death, the appropriateness of resuscitating, even the comparative research approach were adopted from past research. In the early fifties, research articles still referred principally to drowning accidents. The illustrations showed victims (and sometimes rescuers) wearing swimming trunks. The texts[47] discussed drowning at length, but merely mentioned accidents and anesthesiological complications that might lead to sudden death. In surgical settings, researchers implied, mechanical means would be available so that the rescuer need not depend on manual artificial ventilation to reverse the dying process. The principal difference between good and bad technique was the potential to restore artificial ventilation. The emphasis on ventilation was so persistent that the rescuer's energy expenditure was measured in oxygen consumption per unit of time. The choice of a resuscitation method depended on the position, weight, and body type of the victim and on the strength of the rescuer. This variety of guidelines was not considered a problem, as researchers agreed that all artificial-ventilation methods were easy to learn and teach.

How were these techniques implemented? The conference of 1951, where the research groups presented their findings, was attended by representatives of the American National Red Cross, armed forces, Boy Scouts of America, AT&T, Bureau of Mines, Campfire Girls, Girl Scouts of the U.S.A., YMCA, AMA, and public-utility and civil-defense organizations.[48] One major concern of the Red Cross was that the public would lose faith in resuscitation when confronted with a new method. Comroe dismissed this critique when he pointed out that even if the new method saved only 10 percent more lives, the change would be worthwhile. The conference participants decided that they could not afford the confusion that had accompanied the introduction of the Schafer method, in use in the United States by 1909 but not standardized until

1927. To avoid similar confusion, the conferees agreed about a description of the technique. They renamed the method "the back-pressure arm-lift method" (instead of the Nielsen method), so that the name contained the essentials of the technique. They also prepared a two-page standard. These instructions, along with training films, were used in a widespread campaign to teach the back-pressure arm-lift method and limit the Silvester method to special circumstances.

The Obstructed Airway

In 1951, it appeared that the last word about artificial respiration had been written and that the extensive research efforts of the postwar period had identified the "best" resuscitation techniques. But in 1958, several lines of research called for a revision of all manual methods. The main stimulus for change came from Captain Harold Rickard's call for a new manual method for resuscitating small children.

In 1955, Rickard, a captain in the U.S. Navy and a self-proclaimed practitioner of resuscitation for thirty-five years, "invented" a new method for manual artificial respiration in infants and small children. Rickard proposed that different methods be used for children. He also raised the issue of maintaining an open airway. He argued that all recommended resuscitation techniques were useless because even in the face-down position, the airway remained obstructed. The importance of airway clearance was recognized but had not been considered a major problem, in part because researchers had intubated patients for comparison purposes. The intubation had prevented the occurrence of an obstructed airway. Researchers had also kept patients in the face-down position, which made it more difficult to observe the obstruction of the airway.

At a symposium in 1958, Rickard's claim that children needed their own resuscitation technique was rejected for lack of clinical evidence, but indirectly his challenge did influence a revision of resuscitation principles. During the symposium, the anesthesiologist Peter Safar[49] destroyed the myth that patients in the face-down position are less likely to have obstructed airways than those in a face-up position. Armed with new roentgenograms (X rays) and the usual spirometer readings, Safar showed that an obstructed airway is a problem with all manual ventilation methods, regardless of whether the victims are face-up or -down, because an unconscious person's relaxed tongue tends to obstruct the oropharynx. The solution was to hyperextend the neck. Safar strongly recommended the face-up position not only for avoiding the obstruction of the airway but also for increasing the visibility of and accessibility to the victim's face.[50]

This finding was again astonishing. All the research conducted in the fifties had been superseded because the fancy experimental setups had overlooked important field conditions, in this case the obstructed airway. Safar's research was already directed at an alternative technique in the making. His preference for the face-up position and for a method in which one could keep the hands free to check the airway supported mouth-to-mouth resuscitation. Safar's recommendation implied that a century of focusing on manually produced artificial ventilation would need to be abandoned.

Mouth-to-Mouth Ventilation

The origin of mouth-to-mouth ventilation is again the military. In 1950, as part of an army research group, Dick Johns and David Cooper worked on mask-to-mask resuscitation for use on nerve-gas casualties in a contaminated atmosphere. At the beginning of the Korean conflict in 1949, Cooper was called to active duty in the Chemical Corps Medical Laboratories of the Army Chemical Center in Edgewood, Maryland. In mid-March 1950, over beer, Cooper and his roommate Johns discussed the "stupidity"[51] of the U.S. Army and considered what they would change if they had free rein. Cooper mentioned the army's approach to artificial ventilation. He suggested that two gas masks could be linked so that the rescuer's exhaled breath was directed through the lungs of the victim. The next day, the researchers worked on their idea. They removed the leaflet of the victim's exhalation valve, then connected the valves of both masks by a tube with a side arm containing a one-way outlet. They experimented with this device on each other and on some dogs and wrote a report.[52] A week later, they were transferred to other places. Cooper tried to interest the U.S. Navy in their device, but to no avail.

Yet James O. Elam read Johns and Cooper's report. Elam was a young physician who had used mouth-to-mouth ventilation as "an instinctive reflex"[53] when power failures disrupted the iron lungs keeping polio victims alive. In 1950, in his first university position, Elam undertook mouth-to-mouth ventilation research on postoperative patients still under anesthesia with ether. Elam blew in the tracheal tube while two assistants[54] drew blood. His results were vastly superior to those that Gordon's research group had obtained for manual resuscitation.

Elam received an invitation to attend Dill's 1951 conference at the Army Chemical Center in Edgewood, Maryland. Tacked onto the end of the program, Elam was eager to detonate his "bomb." But his presentation on mouth-to-mouth ventilation fizzled: "Whittenberger smiled, Dill yawned, Julius Comroe blinked, and John Clements pointed out that this method, a common sense method, makes it all the more difficult to apply Ted Radford's nomogram."[55] Elam concluded, "One does not overthrow Holger Nielsen (the inventor of the dominant manual artificial ventilation method) and Archer Gordon in a fortnight."[56] He made door-to-door calls to Washington, to the Surgeon General's generals, and to the Red Cross. He also published an article in the *New England Journal of Medicine*[57] and the *American Journal of Physiology*.[58] Even with those publications, Elam did not receive the recognition he hoped for for mouth-to-mouth ventilation. Instead, he was called up for a second round of military duty to the Military Laboratories at Edgewood.

The breakthrough in resuscitation research came in 1956, when Elam received a ride from Safar and his wife from an anesthesiology conference in Kansas. Safar also had used mouth-to-tracheal tube ventilation when inflating patients' lungs after intubation to ascertain bilateral chest movements. By 1956, Safar was in his second year as chief anesthesiologist of Baltimore City Hospitals, and he and Elam set out to compare ventilation volumes produced by manual artificial ventilation with those produced by mouth-to-mouth ventilation. The experiments clearly indicated the superiority of mouth-to-mouth ventilation over manual techniques.

With Elam and Safar's research results in mind, Gordon and his research team[59] embarked on a second comparative study, this time between mouth-to-mouth resuscitation and manual methods. Their results matched those of Elam and Safar. Under all conditions, with endotracheal tube and without, the mouth-to-mouth method was significantly better than the best of the manual ventilation methods. The mouth-to-mouth technique was considered ideal because the face-up position allowed the rescuer to hyperextend the victim's neck and to check for "debris" in the mouth. In 1958, Safar presented his findings at a conference, where participants were also discussing Captain Rickard's suggestion for a new resuscitation method for children. The symposium recommended that "for emergency resuscitation of infants and small children a description of mouth-to-mouth resuscitation, following a preliminary maneuver to clear the airway, should be included in the revised manual."[60] The recommendation that mouth-to-mouth resuscitation be implemented as a complementary method for children is surprising, for in 1948 one of the main objections to the method was that an adult could overinflate the lungs of a smaller victim.[61] The consensus was that "aesthetic aspects precluded a recommendation for direct oral or nasal ventilation of adults."[62] The response among the public and various national and federal organizations was so overwhelming, however, that another ad hoc conference was quickly called to review new research on mouth-to-mouth ventilation in adults. There, mouth-to-mouth (and mouth-to-nose) artificial ventilation techniques became the preferred techniques for all victims; children and adults alike.

In 1960, an international group of researchers tested the mouth-to-mouth resuscitation method in six metropolitan areas in more than 1,000 anesthetized patients and recommended that mouth-to-mouth become the only method to resuscitate all people, with the exception of newborns.[63] They also strongly recommended that the method be taught to both professionals and laypeople. The alternative, promoted by commercial firms, was to insert an oral airway first. The international researchers, however, strongly resisted this commercialism and insisted that the method be simple, safe, and easily learned. The fear of returning to mechanical props prompted the research community to endorse mouth-to-mouth resuscitation for all.

When introducing their "best" resuscitation technique, Safar and Elam lauded the accessibility and visibility of the victim's face to check for the airway and apply mouth-to-mouth ventilation. Because mouth-to-mouth ventilation replaced a century of manual artificial ventilation, they needed to convince potential detractors that the technique was more convenient and efficient than the "theoretical" arguments once invoked to justify resuscitating in the face-down position. Because their new technique was still a form of artificial ventilation, they agreed with their predecessors that death was primarily caused by lack of respiration. Their suggestion to check the airway before artificial ventilation was started did not redefine the dying process. It just made artificial ventilation more effective. And they also continued to link resuscitation with drowning.

Chest Compressions

In 1958, it seemed again that the quest for the best resuscitation technique was complete and that the efforts could now focus on promoting and diffusing mouth-to-mouth ventilation. Only two years later, however, resuscitation research would again shift dramatically when William

Kouwenhoven, Jim Jude, and Guy Knickerbocker developed closed-chest cardiac massage, a simple technique in which the rescuer rhythmically compresses the victim's chest to restore circulation.[64] The reasoning for chest compression was that artificial ventilation alone is useless if oxygenated blood does not reach the brain. Kouwenhoven introduced a different principle: resuscitation required that circulatory function be stimulated. For about two hundred years, the major interventions had been aimed at restoring breathing. Researchers now argued that death was not only a matter of respiration but also of cardiac functions.

Closed-chest cardiac massage developed in the medical laboratories of Johns Hopkins University while the researchers were testing a portable defibrillator, a device that administers electric shocks to reverse a cardiac arrhythmia, called ventricular fibrillation. Instead of a regular beat, the heart in ventricular fibrillation shows a continuous, uncoordinated quivering.[65] If untreated, ventricular fibrillation leads to cardiac arrest, then to clinical death. Ventricular fibrillation can be caused by electric shock. In 1950, the Resuscitation Review Board of the Edison Electric Institute reported that slightly more than 50 percent of fatalities among line workers resulted from ventricular fibrillation, and the institute asked Kouwenhoven, an engineer at Johns Hopkins, to construct a portable defibrillator that could be carried on trucks and used in the field.

While working on the portable closed-chest defibrillator, Knickerbocker, a graduate research assistant, first attempted chest compression. Knickerbocker was testing a prototype of a portable electric defibrillator on dogs when he noticed that the dogs' blood pressure would increase when he put the heavy fifteen-pound paddles of the defibrillator on their chests. Loss of blood pressure was a recurring problem in defibrillator research. After administering an electric shock to throw the heart into ventricular fibrillation, a dog's blood pressure would often drop dramatically before a countershock could be given, causing the animal's death. Knickerbocker and Kouwenhoven had sought ways to maintain the blood pressure, and the pressure of the defibrillator paddles gave Knickerbocker an idea: repeated chest compressions might raise the dogs' blood pressure. In July 1958, with the help of a neighboring laboratory researcher, Dr. Isaacs, Knickerbocker managed to keep a dog alive who had unexpectedly gone into cardiac arrest. The effort lasted for about eight to ten minutes while the defibrillator was retrieved from another floor. Knickerbocker wrote the following note:[66]

Effective external massage was accomplished by method suggested by Dr. Isaacs (exerted force applied to sternum). However, it is very tiring! Mr. Sutton found that standing on the experimental table and massaging with his foot was very effective. In fact, up to eight or ten minutes after fibrillation, the animal had involuntary respiratory movements and eye reflexes in spite of not being defibrillated at all in that interval.

Over the next year, Knickerbocker and Kouwenhoven tested this new practice, which they called "external chest massage." They experimented with different pressures points and compression rates, measured blood flow in the brain, and combined chest compression with the administration of drugs and artificial ventilation. Eventually, they were able to revert five minutes of ventricular fibrillation with external massage. This was a very significant research result. Kouwenhoven's goal was to construct a portable defibrillator and equip every electric-utility truck with it. If "external massage" could gain five minutes, then maybe not all trucks needed to be equipped with defibrillators, or external defibrillation and massage could be combined. The researchers therefore demonstrated their technique to the head of the laboratory, the world-renowned surgeon Dr. Alfred Blalock, who remained skeptical of the technique's efficiency but assigned Dr. James Jude to the project. Jude, a surgeon at Johns Hopkins, could confer medical legitimacy if Knickerbocker and Kouwenhoven were correct.

Jude was impressed with the new resuscitation method for reasons different from the potential benefits for the electric-utility industry. In surgery, cardiac arrest was sometimes an unintended consequence of the administration of anesthesia or invasive surgical procedures. The only solution at the time was to open the patient's chest quickly and put a hand under the heart and massage it by pushing it against the sternum. Surgeons used to carry an extra scalpel in their breast pocket for this purpose. This practice of open-chest cardiac massage often caused serious complications, usually infections. If closed-chest cardiac massage could indeed circulate blood, opening the chest might not be necessary.

Jude attempted the resuscitation method first on a female gallbladder patient whom he admitted from the emergency department. The patient was premedicated and put under anesthesia with a relatively new anesthetic: Halothane. One of the effects of overdosage of Halothane is myocardial depression, which can lead to cardiac arrest. When this patient's tolerance level was exceeded, the anesthesiologist attempted intubation but was unable to ventilate the patient. She became pulseless and cyanotic, and her respiration ceased. When Jude saw the blood pressure and pulse disappear, he put his hands on her chest and started external cardiac massage. No one gave artificial respiration. After two minutes of compressing the chest, a pulse developed, together with spontaneous shallow respirations. A little later, the blood pressure returned, and a new attempt was made at intubation, which eventually succeeded without further cardiac complications. The patient underwent a cholecystectomy and had an uneventful recovery. She was discharged five days later without neurological deficits, and her doctors found her normal on subsequent follow-up examinations.[67]

Jude and his colleagues used closed-chest cardiac massage on four more patients while Knickerbocker and Kouwenhoven continued testing the resuscitation method in the laboratory. On July 9, 1960, the results of the laboratory and clinical research were published in the *Journal of the American Medical Association*. The authors wrote: "Anyone, anywhere, can now initiate cardiac resuscitative procedures. All that is needed are two hands."[68] The shift to cardiac resuscitation was profound, but even more significant was the claim of universality. For the first time, proponents of resuscitation argued that their technology was useful not only for drowning but also for "anyone, anywhere." These words represented one of the most radical shifts in the history of resuscitation research. Anyone could resuscitate, and by implication anyone could be resuscitated. With this new claim to universal resuscitation, all qualifiers that had accompanied resuscitation since the eighteenth century were abandoned. Not only the apparently dead under certain circumstances, but also every dying person, in all conditions, could in principle be revived. Kouwenhoven also offered a new clinical criterion for death. As the absence of a pulse became a sufficient criterion to start chest compression, death became a more refined and clinically palpable transition, a process with gray values. In an article for utility workers, Kouwenhoven wrote, "When a companion, or someone whom you chance to see, falls to the ground, you should run to him [*sic*] and if he is unconscious place him on his back and check for breathing and pulse.... He is in the gray area. It is your responsibility to keep him from slipping beyond it."[69]

How did Kouwenhoven, Jude, and Knickerbocker come to make such a radical claim? These researchers were outsiders, not recipients of the usual resuscitation orthodoxy; their historical ignorance, combined with their familiarity with different audiences, gave them a vantage point from which to make a bold statement.[70] Kouwenhoven's research on electric accidents and defibrillators provided him with enough background to recognize the potential of Knickerbocker's observations. Early in his career, Kouwenhoven had participated in comparative research on the Schafer technique, and although he was familiar with resuscitation research, this was not the engineer's primary research interest. Kouwenhoven's loyalties resided with the utility industry, not with drowning victims. Chest compressions could augment use of the defibrillator because they might bridge the precious minutes that utility workers needed to set up the new instrument. In contrast, Jude's primary audience was other surgeons. Where he was first author, chest compressions were presented as less traumatic than open-heart massage in averting death during surgery.

In addition, the claims of universal resuscitative power also reflected an increasing medicalization of American society. In the golden age of medicine, cumulating after the Second World War, medical drugs and surgical interventions had promised a cure for every disease. Longevity was increasing dramatically; cardiology and cardiac surgery—once considered the last medical frontier—had become a medical specialty; and the birthing and dying processes had solidly become the jurisdiction of medicine. In this context, prolonged mortality for all did not sound like an outrageous promise; instead, it fit the optimistic spirit of the time. Resuscitative techniques also were already applied in a number of life-threatening emergencies. Firefighters and other rescue personnel routinely carried resuscitative apparatus and used it when they thought it appropriate.[71]

Cardiac researchers provided the most radical revision of the resuscitation script since the justification of resuscitation techniques in the eighteenth century. These researchers changed the principle of resuscitation (cardiac instead of ventilation), expanded the number of potential rescuers and potential settings in which their technique could be used, and in the process also redefined the boundaries of human mortality. Drowning victims were no longer the only beneficiaries of resuscitation. Everyone could now aspire to a prolonged life. When mouth-to-mouth ventilation was combined with chest compressions to form CPR (cardiopulmonary resuscitation) at a conference in Maryland in 1960,[72] sudden death was just one more roadblock waiting to be cleared by modern medicine.

THE ORIGINS OF RESUSCITATION BELIEFS

Jude, Kouwenhoven, and Knickerbocker summarized the history of resuscitation research in the following way: "since his origin man [*sic*] has been his brother's keeper. There thus gradually evolved, in modern civilization, the specialized role of the physician or healer who first healed by superstition, then by faith, and finally by science."[73] This familiar modernist tale is historically incorrect. Over time, science and superstition have traded places repeatedly, but faith seems always to be involved in resuscitation. Its history shows that experimentally and clinically "effective" techniques were later abandoned for aesthetic and educational reasons while physiologically "ineffective" techniques saved scores of lives. Mouth-to-mouth ventilation, chest compressions, even defibrillation have been suggested repeatedly as the best means to resuscitate during the past two centuries, but these recommendations were later retracted or denounced. Over a career of resuscitation research, Archer Gordon thought at least twice that he had found the definitive answer, but each time, the technique he had considered best became inferior with new research. Use of improved spirometers retired the popular Schafer method, while a simple laboratory practice, intubating the patient, done to make results comparable, made the manual-ventilation techniques worthless.

New understandings of physiology cannot explain the succession of new techniques. Eventually, each new technique was explained as physiologically more sound, but most were difficult to support on the basis of highest survival rate or the highest yield of oxygen, because these criteria did not lend themselves to easy comparison. With the rapid succession of techniques, survival rates were often unavailable and, if available, failed to discriminate among techniques that seemed to save lives. Previous oxygen yields became irrelevant when research subjects shifted from corpses to hyperventilating volunteers and more precise measuring technology became available. Even when a technique outscored its competitors in dog experiments and in controlled clinical situations there was no guarantee that the technique would be the best in the field. As Dill's research illustrated, even experimental controls that were too strict might fail to identify a useful resuscitation technique. Ultimately, resuscitation has no foolproof criterion; it can be explained only by a unique configuration of social and medical claims.[74] In the next chapter, I explain that medical researchers remain divided on CPR's effectiveness as a resuscitation technique.

In the end, the gradual expansion of faith in efforts to resuscitate emerges along with the technology as the most important achievement over two centuries. Belief in resuscitation grew as the qualifiers that had accompanied lifesaving were abandoned and everyone became implicated in the medicalized process of lifesaving. Instead of an absolute barrier, death became a malleable process. Initially, the Royal Humane Society could deliver its resuscitative promise by making a fine distinction between resuscitating and reanimating and demonstrating that lives in danger at ocean-, lake-, and riverfronts could indeed be saved. But over time, the criteria for a resuscitative effort became more stringent and difficult to achieve. The distinction between reanimating and resuscitating blurred as not only the apparently but also the totally dead became candidates for revival. Next, the criteria for sudden death became narrowly defined to a lack of breathing, later combined with the absence of a pulse. New criteria qualified victims with the barest signs of life as resuscitation candidates. Finally, when Kouwenhoven claimed that "anyone, anywhere" could be revived, not only drowning victims— often young, healthy people—but also all people became candidates for revival. Shifting of definitions thus made the most difficult-to-revive cases, under all circumstances, candidates for CPR.

Kouwenhoven's assertions, however, will remain empty promises until sufficient lives are actually saved. The accepted way to resolve doubt is now to follow CPR in the field and evaluate it with statistical measures such as survival rates. But just as every past technique has come with impressive statistics, statistics in themselves will be insufficient to warrant CPR's adoption. Would it be justifiable to teach CPR to millions if only a small minority of people survive, or do we need survival rates of 50 percent for attempted resuscitative efforts? What counts as a resuscitative effort, anyway, and what counts as survival? Under what circumstances is resuscitating worthwhile? In the next chapter, I will explore how the medical community has rallied behind CPR and turned CPR into a truly universal resuscitation technique, even when its effectiveness, as measured in lives saved, remains unclear.

3   CPR for All

IN THE early sixties, a leading group of resuscitation researchers agreed that CPR—the combination of securing an open airway, mouth-to-mouth ventilation, and chest compressions—was the most promising resuscitation technique. CPR addressed the often fatal problem of an obstructed airway. Further, it incorporated the most successful techniques for artificial ventilation and, for the first time, had the potential to maintain circulation. Important to the reception of CPR was that it did not require props or surgical intervention. It was ideal for both the hospital and the field. Furthermore, it was simple to learn, relatively easy to perform, and not too exhausting. It could be applied quickly, and the laboratory results were favorable. For the enthusiastic believers, CPR's advantages meant that Kouwenhoven's words "anyone, anywhere" should be taken literally. Along with the John Hopkins researchers, they envisioned a world where everyone, from child to elderly adult, would engage in CPR whenever the signs of clinical death loomed.

But when researchers attempted to bridge the gap between a working technique and the outside world, the project for universal CPR met some unexpected problems. Did "anywhere" mean that CPR could be used to save lives both on dirty river banks and in surgery theaters equipped with the latest technology? Did "anyone" imply that not only trained physicians but also paramedics and even laypeople could give chest compressions and mouth-to-mouth ventilation? Each question represented contested terrain previously claimed by other techniques or practitioners. CPR advocates needed to show that the new technique was better, easier, and more efficient than those of the past. In addition, the resuscitation researchers found themselves isolated: their peers in the leading rescue and emergency organizations and in the medical profession did not always share their enthusiasm. Convincing arguments were hard to make when a messy outside world failed to replicate neat laboratory results and when communication problems or a simple traffic jam could foil CPR's lifesaving potential.

At stake was the extent to which CPR was truly universal. Instead of universality in the broadest sense, the leading resuscitation promoters could have opted for a resuscitation system based on an efficacy principle. A CPR system based on efficacy principles required that researchers admit up front that not all deaths could be reversed. They needed to target the deaths with the best chance of reversal—such as electrocution victims. The resuscitative program would thus prove valuable not through quantity of lifesaving for all but through quality of lifesaving for some. Resuscitation would be a specialized activity, and a trained group of professionals would decide whether and when to resuscitate. Universality purists, however, hoped that the sheer quantity of resuscitative efforts would keep survival rates sufficiently high. Some deaths would necessarily slip through the CPR net, but if the mesh were fine enough, numbers of lives could be snatched from the jaws of death.

In the sixties, the efficacy strategy had seemed more feasible than the universality strategy because limiting resuscitation to specific situations followed established traditions. This was a period in which emergency medicine was in its infancy, ambulance systems were underdeveloped, and resuscitation was still associated with drownings and Boy Scout activities. For the first thirteen years of CPR, the technique's scope was indeed limited, but not because its advocates were concerned with its efficacy. Instead, strategists for universality needed more than a decade to make their case. The moral argument for universal CPR needed to be cast in an emergency infrastructure. Only in 1973 did researchers and national rescue organizers design and implement a vast emergency system and embark on an ambitious CPR-training program. By the nineties, CPR had become part of a daily experience, with millions of people trained.

Indiscriminate universal CPR, however, did not save many lives. Survival rates, particularly in big cities, remained disappointingly low. More CPR simply meant that more people died at the end of a resuscitative effort. Only when low survival rates became an undeniable consequence of universal CPR did researchers turn to the question of efficacy, and although they became more aware of the circumstances under which CPR was most effective, they did not act upon this knowledge. Instead of scaling back the technology, the prevailing strategy was to extend the notion of universality further still. Like a gambling habit out of control, universal CPR with low survival rates is the consequence of unrealistic optimism that bigger systems and more techniques will save the most lives.

PROFESSIONAL VERSUS LAY CPR

The first hurdle to universal CPR came from inside the medical world: physicians were reluctant to go along with the notion of lay practitioners. The struggle for universal CPR became a question of whether lifesaving is a medical intervention reserved for health-care professionals or a first-aid technique to be performed by everyone. In 1958, medical organizations agreed that people administering mouth-to-mouth ventilation could do nothing harmful even if they performed the technique unnecessarily and incorrectly.[1] Because of the cardiac component of CPR, however, the situation was different. Physicians in hospitals seized cardiac resuscitation as a medical technique that, if performed inadequately, could cause serious injury. The first years after Kouwenhoven published his findings, pathologists conducting autopsies after failed closed-chest resuscitative attempts reported cracked ribs, ruptured livers, pneumothorax, fractured sternum, bone-marrow emboli, severe hemopericardium, ruptured blood vessels, and other complications.[2] Physicians argued that CPR was too dangerous to be used by the public. They feared that lay rescuers would be unable to define cardiac status before initiating heart compressions. They worried that misdiagnosis would lead to the administration of cardiac resuscitation to, for example, epileptics and people who simply had fainted.[3]

The reports about complications prompted the American Heart Association, the American National Red Cross, and the Industrial Medical Association to issue a warning in 1962 stating that the closed-chest resuscitation method was a *medical* procedure and should be applied only by those who had been carefully trained, such as "physicians, dentists, nurses, and specially qualified emergency rescue personnel."[4] In practice, however, the use of chest compressions was limited to trained physicians. In 1961, Jim Jude, who had become a member of the resuscitation committee of the American Heart Association of Maryland, wrote a handbook about resuscitation.[5] He emphasized the role of nurses in successful resuscitative efforts, noting that they spend more time at the patient's bedside than physicians. The handbook provoked the Maryland State Board of Nurses to warn that nurses should learn the resuscitation technique, but not initiate it. Their task was to assist the physician. In 1961, the medical director of the American Heart Association also issued a memo with a strong warning: "Until further information is available, *heart associations are urged to limit programs on closed-chest cardiac massage to physicians only."* The American Heart Association organized workshops for its physician members but emphasized that these were meant only as a service for practicing physicians, not as an official endorsement of the technique.

The strongest initial resistance to CPR came from within the medical profession. Not only the physicians leading the national rescue organizations but also physicians in primary care, surgeons who had been using open-chest cardiac massage, and emergency department personnel doubted that CPR could deliver on its promises. The disapproval from the major organizations and the reluctance of physicians might have been a severe blow to universal CPR, because limiting chest compressions to physicians defeated the purpose of the technique. Medical professionals and the public at large were aware that physicians could not arrive in time for every cardiac arrest, and all knew that time was the crucial factor in resuscitation. Clearly, more lives would be saved if the public knew the reviving technique. Advocates of universal CPR, however, faced these early setbacks with equanimity. Kouwenhoven was used to skepticism from the medical profession, and his correspondence with other resuscitation advocates shows that he counted on the persuasive power of the resuscitation technique.

Indeed, despite physicians' reluctance to teach CPR to those outside their profession, the general public was intrigued with a simple resuscitation technique that could reverse all sudden deaths. Soon after his publication in 1960, Kouwenhoven received many requests from firefighters and rescue personnel for information and training films about the technique. Kouwenhoven carefully encouraged these people within the boundaries set by the medical profession. He answered requests by pointing out that chest compressions were a medical technique and that lifesaving intervention in the field did not make sense when hospitals were unfamiliar with the method or ill-equipped to care for the patient. He therefore encouraged inquirers to contact physicians and have them order the CPR film, first to train the physicians and hospital authorities, then to teach CPR to rescue squads and firefighters.

The advocates for universal CPR received significant support from people who intuitively believed that CPR would save lives. Several authors conceded that resuscitation techniques had been taught to lay groups without medical supervision. D.T. Clark mentioned the case of a resuscitation "in which massage was performed by a fireman with no instruction."[6] An article about mouth-to-mouth ventilation in Norway indicated that the majority of rescuers had learned the methods from "manuals, folders, newspapers or magazines, or they had heard about it on the radio."[7] At a conference on resuscitation, a Canadian Red Cross delegate confessed that "several labor organizations in Canada have been tempted to jump the gun in teaching this procedure to lay people. Controlling this situation has been a very real problem for us."[8]

In the sixties, physicians straying from the dictum laid down by the American Heart Association and the American National Red Cross provided a more organized attempt to teach resuscitation techniques to laypeople. In 1964, Lois Horvitz, wife of an Ohio publisher, talked during a dinner party with Dr. Claude Beck, a maverick surgeon who had pioneered open-chest defibrillation and was the first to defibrillate a patient successfully. Beck told her about his class on cardiopulmonary resuscitation for physicians. Horvitz attended the class and was convinced that such classes would be beneficial if more people participated. She started the organization Resuscitators of America, Inc., aimed at training lay-people in CPR. By 1966, more than 1,600 people, described by a journalist as "men, women, teenagers, high school coaches, housewives, businessmen, doctors' wives, firemen, cops, and the mayor of a town,"[9] had attended the classes. The organization included chapters in such diverse cities as Altoona, Pennsylvania; Marion, Indiana; Lambertville, New Jersey; Toronto; and San Juan, Puerto Rico. Because it involved laypeople, Resuscitators of America was not recognized by the American Medical Association, and it died out in 1968, a target of the medical organization's concerted efforts to discredit the program.[10]

On the basis of pilot studies and pressure by CPR advocates, however, health-care organizations reclassified the status of CPR in 1965 from a medical procedure to an *emergency* procedure.[11] At this point, the list of potential medical complications was considered "acceptably small" because they were mostly caused by improper implementation. Still, only the actors of 1962—physicians, dentists, nurses, and specially qualified emergency rescue personnel—were allowed to perform CPR. The AMA editorial encouraged the training of nurses and suggested that community hospitals organize resuscitation committees. This recommendation had already been discussed at length with the key advocates of universal resuscitation during the National Health Forum in 1962. Kouwenhoven organized a session with Elam, Gordon, Beck, and Safar, and all agreed that lay CPR was the method of the future, but they decided that they needed to do more preparatory work. Pilot studies had already shown that too quick implementation of CPR could back-fire, especially when hospitals were not prepared to fuel the sparks of life kindled in the outside world. The first need was to equip hospitals with cardiac-arrest programs.

The next year, in 1966, a conference organized by the ad hoc committee on cardiopulmonary resuscitation of the National Research Council did not change the cast of actors involved in CPR. This conference reviewed the existing literature and introduced the "ABC" system of CPR, which designated the sequence of action in a resuscitative effort and also implied a division of labor. Maintaining an airway and performing mouth-to-mouth ventilation to stimulate breathing ("A" and "B") were delegated to nonmedical personnel, while circulation ("C") was the privilege of paramedical personnel. The National Research Council authors also added a "D" for diagnosis, drugs, defibrillation, and disposition[12]—all were exclusive to medical personnel. This division of labor implied that the lay public could perform mouth-to-mouth ventilation but was still not allowed to give chest compressions. Conference proceedings showed that the participants were preoccupied with paving the way for lay CPR by developing a training program. The question-and-answer session reflected this focus:

> Question: How are physicians to be persuaded that certain
>   laypersons should use CPR?
> Dr. Leonard Scherlis: When physicians find that high-risk and
>   paramedical groups in their communities are being taught
>   CPR, they become more willing to extend this teaching to
>   others.... In terms of priority, the physicians should be taught
>   first, then the allied health care professions and paramedical
>   personnel, as we have indicated. Sometimes physicians do
>   not accept these suggestions until they are "pressured" by
>   other groups in the area or until medico-legal considerations
>   make it increasingly necessary for them to become expert in
>   these measures.[13]

Scherlis's answer underscored the resistance to CPR within the medical profession. Physicians needed some legal arm-twisting to learn the new resuscitation method. To Scherlis and the other CPR advocates, universal CPR seemed inevitable. Timing, however, was important. The conference members conceded that there simply were not enough instructors to teach this method to the general public. They also requested more pilot studies.

When those studies became available, they showed that the general public could learn CPR and perform it as adequately as medical professionals. CPR was thus a relatively safe procedure. The unanswered question was the number of lives that would be saved through public participation in CPR. The results of the scattered pilot studies were not promising: survival rates remained low. Privately, some loyal advocates of universal CPR expressed dissatisfaction with the low survival rates and looked for ways to perk them up. In a letter to a friend in the utility industry, for example, Kouwenhoven expressed his concern: "I am worried about the lack of success we are having with heart–lung resuscitation. I should like to have your suggestions as to what we can do to improve the record. Your men are in good health, as a rule, and I believe that better results can be obtained. What can I do? What have I failed to do? This situation concerns me."[14] Kouwenhoven consequently focused on mechanical ventilators used in the utility industry. He reasoned that these devices voided the effect of CPR. Thus, while resuscitation researchers knew early about the method's low survival rates, they did not question its principles. Instead, they looked for improvements that could enhance survival.

PATIENT TRANSPORTATION

The pilot studies also indicated that CPR's reviving benefits could be improved if lifesaving actions were followed by quick transportation to the hospital. Hearts restarted in the field required intensive monitoring and follow-up, and often additional surgery in a hospital setting. Until the mid- to late sixties, emergency transportation was erratic at best. Independent of the push for universal CPR, however, the ambulance system was reorganized during this period, and universal CPR took advantage of a reorganized system of emergency management.

Before reorganization, the closest doctor, hospital-based ambulance personnel, or firefighters attended victims of accidents or the patient was transported to the hospital using a pushcart, delivery wagon, or coach. A number of urban hospitals in cities such as Cincinnati, New York, and Philadelphia had maintained ambulance services since 1865, and these ambulances transported patients to hospitals or their homes when police officers warned hospitals via telegraph or telephone. First-aid texts for ambulances were rare, and military texts on battlefield medicine were adapted for emergency medicine in civilian accidents. A surgeon, driver, and gatekeeper responded to the call. Other cities, including Albany, Detroit, St. Louis, and Chicago, did not maintain regular ambulance service.[15]

Most cardiac-arrest cases ended up in the "DOA," or "dead on arrival," category. The sociologist David Sudnow conducted ethnographic research in two EDs in 1962–63 and described the interaction between ambulance personnel and doctors with regard to DOA patients:

> When an ambulance driver suspects that the person he is carrying is dead, he signals the Emergency Ward with a special siren alarm as he approaches the entrance driveway. As he wheels his stretcher past the clerk's desk, he restates his suspicion with the remark, "possible," a shorthand reference for "possible DOA." The clerk records the arrival in a logbook and pages a physician, informing him, in code, of the arrival. The "person" is rapidly wheeled to the far end of the ward corridor and into the nearest available foyer, supposedly out of sight of other patients and possible onlookers of the waiting room. The physician arrives, makes his examination, and pronounces the patient dead, or not.[16]

Sudnow added that "it is interesting to note that while the special siren alarm is intended to mobilize quick response on the part of the ER staff, it occasionally operates in the opposite fashion. Some ER staff came to regard the fact of a DOA as decided in advance; they exhibited a degree of nonchalance in answering the siren or page, taking it that the 'possible DOA' most likely is a 'D.'" In addition to ambulance services, fire departments in some cities offered first-aid and mechanical resuscitation, but they were not equipped to transport patients. Inadequate attention to emergency transportation caused a presidential commission on highway safety in 1966 to decry the many deaths during traffic accidents as a "neglected disease of society." Out of the commission came a national curriculum for emergency medical technicians.

Patient transportation moved into a new phase in 1966, when J. Frank Pantridge and John Geddes at the Royal Victoria Hospital in Belfast, Ireland, organized the first mobile intensive-care unit staffed with an ambulance driver, a physician, and a nurse. They knew from the published literature and personal experience that people younger than fifty-five died within an hour of onset of cardiac-arrest symptoms, while admission to the hospital was often delayed for more than twelve hours. In an attempt to ensure quick and safe transportation of patients, they equipped an old ambulance with a defibrillator and developed a protocol for emergency response. When a patient suffered cardiac arrest, onlookers would first contact the family physician. If physicians suspected a heart attack, they called an easy-to-memorize hospital emergency number. The hospital operator warned the ambulance driver, who picked up the physician and nurse. Usually within fifteen minutes, the ambulance reached the patient's house. After a year of sending out the ambulance, not one of the first 312 patients had died in transit, and 155 had been diagnosed with a myocardial infarction. Ten patients were resuscitated outside the hospital; five of those were discharged alive.[17]

In 1967, Pantridge and Geddes published their experience with the mobile intensive-care unit in the prestigious British medical journal *The Lancet*, and within two years, the program was copied in Europe, Australia, and the United States. Although several U.S. programs first placed physicians in ambulances, deploying M.D.s was soon deemed too expensive, and organizers opted instead for paramedic ambulance crews. Most programs worked with firefighters who traditionally had been summoned for rescues, resuscitations, and accidents. Inspired by Pantridge, physicians upgraded the ambulances with equipment—an electrocardiograph, a defibrillator, a supply of oxygen, and cardiac drugs. Eager to show the best results with the invigorated ambulance systems, the doctors trained their staff in CPR and basic patient-assessment skills. But it soon became apparent that even with better emergency response, the success of these first programs in reversing sudden death was mixed. In an experiment in Brookline, Massachusetts, for example, emergency physicians developed a three-session training course for police and fire-department rescue personnel. The emphasis was on the criteria for identifying cardiac arrest, precautions to avoid injuries, and the need to combine chest compressions with assisted breathing. Of the first twenty-five resuscitative efforts, only one patient survived. The lone survivor was exceptional because he had collapsed at a party where a fire chief, recently trained in CPR, was present.

Legal issues created other obstacles in the field. One was rescuers' failure to move patients to the hospital, where a defibrillator and drugs could be used. The principal reason for delay was the uncertainty over whether the person was alive or dead, as the law prohibited moving a dead body without authorization. Researchers also had to confront the hierarchy of command. They found that for firefighters, while the initiation of the resuscitation procedure was the responsibility of the officer in charge, the decision to move the patient was made by a deputy chief, usually someone untrained in cardiac resuscitation and unaware of the urgency. Important time was thus lost in administration. Another complication was that most local physicians were unfamiliar with CPR and terminated the resuscitation attempt, regardless of whether a rescuer's efforts seemed effective. Researchers also discerned a marked difference between firefighters and police. The police, who were usually first at the scene of the accident or fire, were less likely to initiate resuscitation. Many were apprehensive about the possibility of legal liability and expressed a fear of exposure to contagious disease. The solution was to equip police squad cars with bag and mask resuscitators.

More equipment and better-integrated systems became the goals of ambulance advocates, whose anecdotal accounts did not always mask the ongoing problem with survival rates. In Miami, the anesthesiologist Eugene Nagel experimented with physicians monitoring defibrillation by radio while paramedics followed instructions in the field. In 1970, Nagel reported the following case study:

> A 68 year-old woman had been talking to her family when she collapsed. Fire Rescue arrived on the scene three minutes after receipt of the alarm and immediately commenced emergency ventilation and circulation. The telemetry electrodes were attached to the patient and an ECG transmitted. Fire Rescue was advised that the patient was in ventricular fibrillation and was requested to transmit a confirmatory ECG. After receipt of the second ECG, which confirmed ventricular fibrillation, Rescue was advised to defibrillate. Following a single defibrillation at 400 watt seconds a third ECG transmission was made. On the basis of this last transmission the hospital doctor advised Rescue that the victim was successfully defibrillated and to continue resuscitation. Fire Rescue accompanied the patient in the ambulance to the hospital, monitoring ECG and vital signs on the way. During this time the pupillary response was good and the patient occasionally attempted voluntary respiration. The patient's hospital course was marred by repeated cardiac arrhythmias resulting in her death on the seventh hospital day.[18]

In 1969, the Seattle physician Leonard Cobb and fire chief Gordon Vickery proposed a two-tiered response system. A first-aid unit initially responded to the call, followed by a mobile intensive-care unit staffed with paramedics trained in defibrillation and IV care. In 1972, Cobb also initiated one of the first lay CPR programs when he organized the teaching, reportedly, of more than 500,000 citizens.

The success rate in lives saved by those first programs was relatively low. In Baltimore, the rate was 10 percent; in Brookline, Massachusetts, it was 4 percent. Mobile coronary-care units in New York City made 161 calls, finding nineteen patients with serious heart disease and three with ventricular fibrillation; only one was successfully resuscitated.[19] In Los Angeles, of ninety-three patients found with ventricular fibrillation, twelve became long-term survivors.[20] Directors of paramedic programs did not consider these numbers low because they were considered still better than past alternatives and because the shortened transportation time suggested grounds for optimism. Although physicians in metropolitan centers expressed concern about traffic congestion, they reasoned that shortening the transportation time combined with greater community sensitivity would eventually propel survival rates upward.

CONSOLIDATION OF THE EMERGENCY MEDICAL SYSTEM

In 1973, thirteen years after the method of closed-chest cardiac massage was first described in the *Journal of the American Medical Association*, a National Conference on Standards for CPR and Emergency Cardiac Care (ECC) recommended the integration of universal lay CPR with the emerging paramedic-based ambulance systems. The result was the laying out of an emergency medical-care system that would address sudden death comprehensively. With Archer Gordon as chair, the conference participants distinguished between basic and advanced lifesaving intervention. Basic life support was CPR; it should be taught to everyone. Advanced life support went further to encompass use of adjunctive equipment, intravenous fluid lifelines, drug administration, defibrillation, stabilization of the victim via cardiac monitoring, controlling of arrhythmias, and post-resuscitation care. Advanced cardiac life support was reserved for specially trained health-care professionals. To achieve universal CPR, conferees agreed, the general public needed to be taught the technique and educated about the risk factors that can lead to a heart attack and the related early-warning signs.[21] Initially, groups with the greatest needs, such as police officers, firefighters, rescue workers, lifeguards, high-risk industrial workers, and families of cardiac patients, received preference, but the goal was to train the public, starting with schoolchildren at the eighth-grade level. The American Heart Association decided to standardize and disseminate CPR protocols and organize the training and certification of instructors (see Figure 3-1). In addition, primary-care physicians needed to familiarize themselves with the emergency systems in their communities.

To implement advanced life support comprehensively, the conference participants proposed a three-level system of coronary care. The

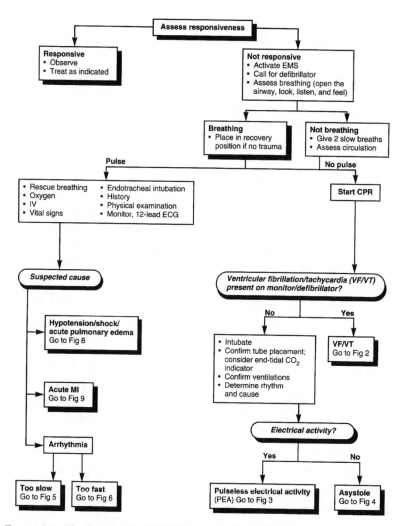

FIGURE 3-1. The Standardized CPR Protocol. (Reproduced with permission, *Advanced Cardiac Life Support*, 1997. Copyright American Heart Association.)

first level consisted of life-support units and included anyone trained in CPR. Advanced care was performed by the paramedic-staffed mobile life-support units and by the staff of hospital EDs. The guidelines specified necessary equipment and drugs and provided suggestions for ambulance design. The second level of the system involved hospital-based coronary-care units. Coronary care was initially instituted to provide intensive postoperative monitoring for cardiac patients, many of whom died after successful operations. After coronary-care units were implemented, advocates claimed that the mortality rate dropped by as much as one-third, largely because of the contributions of specially trained coronary-care nurses.[22] The conference organizers suggested expanding the mandate of these popular units to encompass monitoring patients in the acute phase of a heart attack or in post-resuscitative care. The third level, consisting of regional reference centers, was not explained in the 1973 guidelines.

The thirty-two-page final document did not predict how many lives would be saved through this massive investment of human power and resources, but this omission was not deliberate. Swept away by positive findings and widespread optimism, the conference organizers simply assumed that with public CPR and a vast emergency medical system in place, a significant number of lives would be saved. Most believed that any saved life was better than a sudden death. But the architects of the system glossed over several unresolved problems. First, neither CPR nor new systems of patient transportation had resulted in dramatic lifesaving advances. Second, in their struggle to get everyone to resuscitate, advocates of universal CPR failed to consider that not every patient in cardiac arrest is a good candidate for a resuscitative intervention. By the early seventies, medical researchers had already become aware of the two main factors influencing survival: speed of resuscitative care and underlying cardiac etiology.[23] Those with certain cardiac dysrhythmias, such as asystole, had almost no chance of survival, while those with ventricular fibrillation had a much better prognosis. Researchers in Belfast had noted in 1969 that twenty-seven of forty-eight patients in ventricular fibrillation had survived cardiac arrest, while none of the fifty-eight patients in asystole had survived.[24] This finding meant that CPR was not indicated for every sudden death; rather, it worked only under particular conditions. But researchers disregarded differences in survival based on cardiac rhythm, even though they could seriously depress survival rates. The other factor explaining success, a speedy response, became the theme of resuscitative care. The Belfast researchers had demonstrated that the chances for recovery dwindled to negligible after the "window of opportunity" closed; this critical period was the four to six minutes after the first signs of clinical death occurred. The 1973 conference organizers hoped that more advanced technology might soon tackle the problem of asystole or open a wider "window of opportunity" and push back the boundaries of unexpected death even farther.

Although the guidelines lacked cohesion, the goal of emergency planning was clear. Every sudden death had become an unwanted death. As conference organizers wrote, "unless otherwise indicated, these standards are universally applicable."[25] Counter-indications consisted of a single sentence, buried in an upbeat medico-legal section assuring the need for legal Good Samaritan coverage for people administering resuscitative care in good faith: "Cardiopulmonary resuscitation is not indicated in certain situations, such as in cases of terminal irreversible illness where death is not unexpected or where prolonged cardiac arrest dictates the futility of resuscitation efforts."[26] Advocates further included energetic calls for pro-resuscitation legislative action, making CPR the center of a new emergency medical system and turning resuscitative care into a standard operating procedure. From first responder to paramedic to ED to coronary-care unit, the goal was to save, in Claude Beck's words, "hearts too good to die."[27] As the organizers intended them, the guidelines formed the blueprint for doctors and regional heart associations to set up emergency medical systems, to lobby politicians, and to mobilize professional and government organizations. More than five million copies of the 1973 guidelines, in several languages, were distributed worldwide along with materials for teaching CPR, primarily developed by the American Heart Association and the American National Red Cross. These organizations began teaching hundreds of thousands of Americans the "ABCs" of lifesaving. CPR had arrived as a universal resuscitation technique in the United States.

SURVIVAL RATES

Yet survival rates remained unexamined once an emergency infrastructure was firmly in place and the start-up problems had been ironed out. Even today, a general, comprehensive CPR survival rate for the United States is unavailable. There is no national registry (such as the cancer and cystic fibrosis registries),[28] no national database, no governmental or nongovernmental organization that centralizes information on a national level to track the success or failure of resuscitative attempts. Medical researchers and policymakers do not know how many people are treated with CPR and ACLS, and they do not know how many survive. The main indicator of CPR's effectiveness is a plethora of regional survival rates based on short-term, small-scale studies. These rates tend to vary enormously, as Mickey Eisenberg and his colleagues[29] found when analyzing the survival rates in twenty-nine cities in the United States and abroad between 1967 and 1988. They came up with a wide diversity of rates, ranging from 2 percent in Iowa to 26 percent in King County, Washington.

Taken together, the survival rates that these small studies reported provided a sobering picture and confirmed the suspicions of many ED staff. CPR and the emergency infrastructure had not reversed as many sudden deaths as the 1973 conference participants had hoped. The general public had indeed learned CPR and had become sensitized to the signs of cardiac arrest because in several communities half the resuscitative efforts began with bystander response. Most communities had also implemented ambulance systems, some staffed with volunteers, others with professionals; some of them EMTs, others paramedics or firefighters. Some communities had only one layer of rescue care; others had implemented a tiered system. But whatever the system, the point of diminishing return in survival was reached quickly. The average age of patients who had been resuscitated, which ranged from fifty-eight to seventy, indicated the drawbacks of universality. CPR was used indiscriminately. Any death had become a potential candidate for resuscitative intervention. The result was a disappointingly low survival rate.

Still, a new generation of researchers in the nineties attempted to figure out what made the difference between a rate of 2 percent and one of 26 percent. The numbers implied that in Iowa, one in fifty resuscitative efforts is successful, whereas in Seattle, one in four results in saving a life. But to make sense of those numbers, resuscitation in Seattle and Iowa should be similar events, and when Eisenberg attempted a comparison, major methodological and terminological differences appeared. For example, one recognized variable that might influence survival after cardiac arrest is the time between the patient's collapse and the initiation of the resuscitative efforts, often called response time. Eisenberg noted that the literature provided no clear definition of response time:

> [T]he term "response time" may involve all or some of the following: recognition time, decision to call time, calling time, dispatch interview time, dispatching time, time from station to arrival at scene, and time from scene to arrival at patient's side. In addition to response time, variations in definitions exist for such basic terms as cardiac arrest, bystander CPR, witnessed arrest, V[entricular] F[ibrillation], and admission.[30]

Even more significant for comparison was that researchers defined the two key components of a survival rate—resuscitation and survival—differently. Some limited a resuscitative effort to particular cardiac rhythms, such as ventricular tachycardia; others included any attempt at CPR as a resuscitative effort. Survival was also a very ambiguous concept. In some cities, it meant that patients were discharged alive from the hospital with minimal neurological damage; in others, it referred to admission to the intensive-care unit with a viable pulse, a criterion that included comatose patients. The interpretation of regional survival rates was further confounded by differences within and between emergency systems, by varying quality of the programs, and by dissimilar demographic characteristics of the population. This methodological potpourri rendered the regional survival rates incomparable and incomprehensible.

The terminological "Tower of Babel"[31] overshadowing survival rates prompted the Utstein consensus conference on a small island off the Norwegian coast in 1991. There an international task force recommended a template approach for data reporting, attempted to define the terms of a resuscitative effort, set standards for temporal intervals, and suggested a uniform formula for the calculation of the survival rate (see Figure 3-2).[32] Although the Utstein guidelines constituted a remarkable standardization, the conference did not calculate a comprehensive national survival rate. One optimistic commentator suggested that an overall survival rate was no longer necessary: "The Utstein style is a clear reminder that system outcomes limited to survival rates are out of date."[33] With the template approach, measuring the outcome was not limited to who lives or dies; it made possible more fine-grained measures. In certain cases, resuscitative intervention could still be "cost-effective," depending on the longevity and the survivor's functioning, and rates could reflect a more nuanced definition of survival.[34]

The Utstein guidelines formed an important step in determining after twenty-three years why and how CPR works well in some communities and less well in others. Some medical researchers admitted that in the past "the cart was put before the horse,"[35] and they wanted to set the scientific record straight. But even the template approach allowed only a limited number of questions, slanted in a particular direction. For example, what did the survival rate measure, and what was excluded from measurement? Although the Utstein members did not calculate a survival rate for the United States, they provided a standard definition

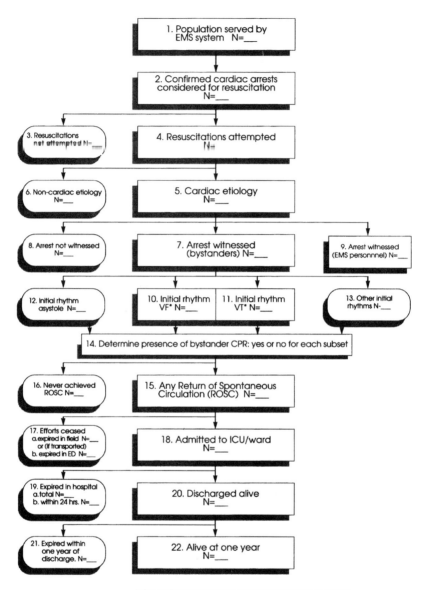

*VF and VT should be reported separately through template

FIGURE 3-2. The Utstein Template for Out-of-Hospital Resuscitation Data. (Reproduced with permission, *Recommended Guidelines for Uniform Reporting of Data From Out-of-Hospital Cardiac Arrest: The Utstein Style,* 1991. Copyright American Heart Association.)

to be used in future studies: "the number [of patients] discharged alive [from the hospital] divided by the number of persons with witnessed cardiac arrest, in ventricular fibrillation, of cardiac etiology."[36]

This standard Utstein survival rate included only a small proportion of attempted resuscitative efforts. Only an underlying cardiac etiology qualified a resuscitative endeavor for inclusion in the statistics, and some of the incidents and accidents that over the past two centuries had made up the most common conditions for resuscitative intervention were written out. Sudden infant death syndrome, drug overdose, suicide, hypoxia, exsanguination, cerebrovascular accidents, subarachnoid hemorrhage, trauma, and—surprisingly—drownings were all conditions resulting from non-cardiac etiologies. Although the same lifesaving sequences would be performed on these victims, and although they had been included in some regional statistics, they were excluded from the Utstein survival rate. Also excluded were unwitnessed cardiac arrest, patients without initial ventricular tachycardia or ventricular fibrillation, and patients on whom bystanders did not initially perform CPR. Because only cases with the best possible chance of survival were eligible for inclusion, the survival rate was inflated when compared with studies using a more comprehensive definition. Instead, most conditions prompting CPR were not included in the statistics. Early studies indicated that 61–80 percent of instances of attempted CPR were excluded from the calculations, presumably because these situations lacked a good chance for survival.[37]

Counteracting this best possible sample, however, was the requirement that the patient be discharged alive from the hospital. This criterion created a relatively high standard for survival in resuscitative efforts, but it too lacked uniformity. Throughout the United States and certainly around the world—the criteria used to discharge patients differed significantly. So did assumptions regarding disability. Although only patients "discharged alive" counted as survivors, a post–Utstein researcher wrote that "individuals whose level of neurological function required transfer to a chronic care facility were coded as non-survivors."[38] People who are institutionalized are thus considered non-survivors; for statistical purposes, those with neurological disabilities are considered dead.

The Chain of Survival

Since 1991, a few local studies have calculated survival rates according to the Utstein template, and the results have not been spectacularly different from the pre–Utstein studies. Although they were based on the healthiest and most homogeneous sample possible, survival rates remained generally low and still varied tremendously. For example, in a follow-up study of 2,071 cardiac-arrest cases in New York City, 415 qualified according to the Utstein criteria.[39] The overall survival rate was 1.4 percent; the survival rate of the subgroup was 5.3 percent. In Oakland County, Michigan, a research group analyzed 2,152 arrests of presumed cardiac origin, and only 476 met the Utstein criteria.[40] Of this subsample, 14.9 percent were discharged alive. In Charlotte, North Carolina, 39 percent of 627 patients fit the Utstein criteria. Survival to discharge was accomplished in 5 percent of the subsample.[41] The Utstein-approved group of patients left Chicago researchers with only 22 percent of their sample of 6,451 patients, and the survival rate for this subgroup was 3.5 percent. Taking all resuscitative attempts into account, the researchers found a bleak survival rate of 0.8 percent for African Americans and 2.6 percent for Caucasians in Chicago.[42] The Chicago researchers aptly titled their article "Outcome of CPR in a Large Metropolitan Area—Where Are the Survivors?"

How were those rates interpreted? The medical literature was consistently optimistic. This consistency was not surprising, considering that, as a critic remarked,[43] about 85 percent of all CPR-related research articles in the United States came from a community of ten research groups. Those groups included the same people who agreed on the CPR protocols, decided on the Utstein criteria, advised the American Heart Association, belonged to editorial boards, and presumably peer-reviewed each other's work. According to this research community, the best possible resuscitation rates could be obtained in any "mature"[44] emergency systems with the appropriate infrastructure and political will power. The low survival rates that plagued most of the less "mature" emergency systems—including those in most major metropolitan areas—in the United States were, according to the dominant view, temporary aberrations. The most widely cited survival rates were obtained from Seattle and suburban King County, Washington. Based on the most favorable subsample and intensive CPR promotion campaigns, those studies yielded much higher survival rates (30%)[45] than the rest of the country. In a defense to the incredulity he faced when presenting his data (his colleagues wondered whether the ubiquitous moss in Seattle was cardio-protective), Eisenberg argued that Seattle and King County were "simply able to deliver CPR, defibrillation, and advanced care rapidly," and he claimed that his example of "the perfect resuscitation" could have happened in any community with an identical outcome.[46] For now, with the exception of a tiny island community in the Pacific Northwest, no community has ever come close to replicating the Seattle–King County experience.[47]

Eisenberg's editorial set the tone for the way most post–Utstein survival rates, however high or low, were analyzed. Higher survival rates would follow, analysts assumed, if we strengthened the four links of the chain of survival. In 1991, the importance of community-based resuscitative care was confirmed when the American Heart Association adopted this simple concept. The chain of survival had four major interdependent links: early access, early basic CPR, early defibrillation, and early ACLS. If any of the links in the chain were inadequate, the result would be less-than-optimal survival (see Figure 3-3). The chain of survival not only defined the standard sequence for resuscitative care; it has also become an interpretative standard. For example, Lance Becker, who found the dismal 0.8 percent survival rate for African Americans in Chicago, remained unwavering in his belief in the four links of the emergency medical system: "Given the low survival rates observed, it is *logical* that improving the links in the chain of survival for all victims will result in a substantial improvement in the survival rates for blacks."[48] The New York researchers, who reported a survival rate of slightly more than one out of one hundred out-of-hospital cardiac arrests, provided similar recom-

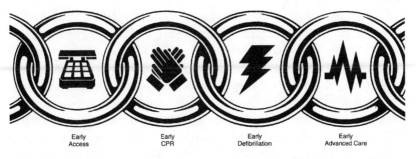

| Early Access | Early CPR | Early Defibrillation | Early Advanced Care |

FIGURE 3-3. The Four Links of the Chain of Survival. (Reproduced with permission, *Improving Survival from Sudden Cardiac Arrest*, 1991. Copyright American Heart Association.)

mendations: "We feel that the most effective way to improve survival rates in New York City is to train other uniformed services as first responders. Adding first responders with defibrillation capabilities offers the possibility of strengthening the first three links in the chain of survival: early access, early CPR, and early defibrillation."[49] Because significant factors for survival—the type of cardiac dysfunction and a witness to the arrest—remain out of direct control, medical commentators focused on system-related factors: a rapid response time, automatic defibrillators for EMTs, better lay training, follow-up programs,[50] and the discontinuation of failed resuscitative efforts in the ED.[51] In the most critical analysis I could find in a major medical journal, an article entitled, "Unsuccessful Emergency Medical Resuscitation—Are Continued Efforts in the Emergency Department Justified?" researchers in Rhode Island showed that the total cost to the hospital for the sixteen (out of 185) patients admitted to the intensive-care unit was $180,908, and that *none* of the patients had survived to be discharged from the hospital. But the researchers still concluded that we should not give up on CPR: "Specifically, measures should be taken to increase the number and responsiveness of emergency medical units capable of defibrillation, performed either by trained paramedics or with automatic external defibrillators, and to provide widespread instruction for lay-people in techniques of cardiopulmonary resuscitation, since these are the two modifiable determinants of survival."[52] This conclusion was contradicted by the presented research findings and reflected the prevalent preconceptions in the resuscitation field. These studies have shown convincingly and repeatedly that universal resuscitative efforts have only minor lifesaving effects, which quickly level off, and that improvements require huge investments.

Of the four links in the "chain of survival," early defibrillation has become the golden link that, researchers assert, will miraculously increase survival rates. The reasoning behind the push for defibrillators was that researchers agreed (albeit reluctantly and implicitly) that survival rates based on CPR alone were negligible. But the chances for survival were better if patients in ventricular fibrillation were targeted for resuscitative attempts. Some studies indicated that 80–90 percent of survivors had been treated for ventricular fibrillation.[53] Current strategy is therefore to promote the widespread availability of defibrillators, and CPR advocates are envisioning a society in which the defibrillator is standard equipment of airplanes, health clubs, offices, street corners, and homes, much as fire extinguishers and smoke detectors are now. The newest generation of defibrillators are "semi-automatic," so that once the electrodes are connected and a button is pushed, the machine reads the cardiac rhythm and, if fibrillation has occurred, shocks the patient after sounding a warning. No special training is required to handle the machine.

Do defibrillators save more lives? When defibrillators were introduced in King County, Washington, the survival rate for patients in ventricular fibrillation increased from 7 percent to 26 percent.[54] Survival rates in California increased from negligible numbers to 13 percent when automatic defibrillators were made available to emergency medical technicians.[55] In some Wisconsin communities, the survival rate rose from 3.6 percent to 6.4 percent for all cardiac arrests, and was 11 percent for patients initially in ventricular fibrillation.[56] Other studies in Pittsburgh, Pennsylvania; Memphis, Tennessee; and Charlotte, North Carolina, however, have shown that adding automatic external defibrillators to the emergency medical system has not significantly improved the chances of survival from cardiac arrest.[57] The authors of a recent study caution that, "as an isolated enhancement, it is doubtful that addition of AED [automated external defibrillator] will provide a measurable survival benefit."[58] Others have been more blunt: "many of the cardiac arrest patients did not require this intervention [defibrillation], and, even if they did, most still failed to survive. In fact, the majority never even achieved restoration of spontaneous circulation."[59] Although much unexplored difference remains between regions, and the number of saved lives seems to plateau quickly, the infinitely optimistic emergency community has chosen to ignore signs that the effectiveness of automatic defibrillating may be limited (they now add the caveat that the focus on defibrillation should not lead to a weakening of the other links in the chain of survival). Instead, indiscriminate defibrillation is promoted as a way to achieve immortality. Pushing the hype a little further, a lawyer has warned emergency system directors that they may be liable if they do not offer defibrillation as part of standard out-of-hospital resuscitative care.[60]

Some CPR Is Better Than No CPR

Not surprisingly, the Utstein guidelines are not aimed at figuring out *whether* CPR (and ACLS) is effective. CPR has remained the only accepted way to resuscitate patients. Improvements have been possible, but alternatives have not. Richard Cummins, who initiated the Utstein conference and promoted the chain-of-survival concept, wrote explicitly in 1995: "Now researchers must shift from a longstanding interest in how and whether CPR works. We must now focus on improving CPR techniques, making CPR work better, getting more people to learn CPR, and getting more people to start CPR."[61] In a paradigm in which the value of CPR is beyond question, survival rates have become a *post factum* justification; data provide guidelines for tinkering but not for overhauling the system.[62] This sentiment was confirmed in 1992 when the American Heart Association adopted the principle that "some CPR is better than no CPR," meaning that even badly performed CPR is better than no CPR at all.

At the same time that the researchers have taken CPR for granted, they remain skeptical that CPR alone can reverse sudden death. The resuscitative efforts in which the patient recover at the scene after bystanders performed CPR are dismissed for statistical purposes as "near-arrests." Researchers apparently do not believe that CPR alone is ever sufficient to reverse sudden death. They assume instead that the rescuer did not assess the patient correctly and that the situation was not a true cardiac arrest but one in which the patient had a difficult-to-palpate pulse, was in a deep sleep, or had experienced a similarly non–life-threatening mishap.

So why do medical researchers still recommend CPR? Basically, CPR needs to keep the body viable enough for rescuers to arrive with an electric defibrillator. A variety of international studies have indicated that patients who undergo early CPR are more likely to have ventricular fibrillation. The Belgian Cardio-Pulmonary-Cerebral Resuscitation Registry, for example, reported a 42 percent prevalence of ventricular fibrillation when patients in cardiac arrest were given bystander CPR, compared with 29 percent in patients given delayed CPR.[63] CPR is viewed as a weak temporary measure to keep the patient in the best possible heart rhythm until a defibrillator is available.

The current survival rates are thus part of a scientific story in which the assumptions, the interpretation, and the conclusion are predetermined. Only the numbers need to be plugged in, and it does not really matter how high or low the numbers are. Emergency researchers are convinced that CPR and the community-based emergency system work. All the bets are now on showing how much survival improves with electric defibrillation. If the numbers are low, it means that we need to strengthen the emergency infrastructure and cover the streets with defibrillators. If the numbers are high (coincidentally, the numbers obtained in the area where the leading resuscitation researchers reside), we have a "mature" emergency medical system, exemplars for others. The Utstein survival rate is constructed to make these points loud and clear.

What Is Survival?

The Utstein criteria defined survival as live hospital discharge, but when emergency staff are resuscitating a patient, they do not know whether he or she will actually be discharged alive. Even when a patient is stabilized and transferred to the intensive-care unit, he or she might be discharged alive, die, or experience neurological impairment and be transferred to a long-term nursing institution. How many patients are in this last category? The information is very sketchy. In Chicago, Lance Becker noted, 519 patients (out of 6,451 cardiac-arrest patients) were transferred to the intensive-care unit. Of those, 108 left the hospital, but we do not know what happened to the remaining 411 patients. In King County, Washington, a group of 150 patients in either asystole or EMD[64] were admitted to the hospital, but only thirteen of them left the hospital. No information is available about the other 137 patients. In Michigan, Robert Swor reported that of 183 (of 722 witnessed, unmonitored out-of-hospital cardiac arrests admitted to the hospital), seventy-six patients were discharged alive. Nothing is said about the majority of the 107 other patients.[65] William Gray noted that of the sixteen patients admitted to the hospital in the Rhode Island study, none survived to the point of discharge. One patient regained consciousness, but died the same day. Another remained in a comatose condition for four months.[66]

A cautious conclusion we can draw from these studies is that the number of people who remain in the hospital after being stabilized is several times higher than the number of patients who are discharged alive. But in most cases, we do not know whether the people admitted to the hospital died or whether they remained in a permanent vegetative state. For that matter, we know nothing about the cognitive functioning of those who are discharged alive. Can they resume their previous lives, or are they severely neurologically incapacitated? An observer concluded, "The information about the quality of life of those who survived CPR after circulatory arrest is scarce and usually restricted to subjective observations in the margin of studies that have for their object the survival after CPR."[67]

Indeed, the resuscitation research community has been quiet about what "discharged alive with no or minimal neurological damage" actually means and what happens to people who are transferred to the intensive-care unit but do not walk out of the hospital. A follow-up study of thirty patients admitted to a hospital in Innsbruck, Austria, offers a rare view of the different shades of survival:

> Thirteen of the 30 resuscitated patients survived and were discharged from the ICU after a mean [stay] of 16.2 days. At the final clinical neurological examination four weeks after admission, six of them (46.2%) presented with good cerebral performance (consciousness, alertness, and the ability to work and lead a normal life). In five patients (38.5%) moderate cerebral disability was found: two of them suffered from a slight hemiparesis, one patient developed generalized seizures, and two patients exhibited memory deficits and mental changes. One patient survived with severe cerebral disability, suffering from cortical blindness, hemiplegia, seizures, and severe memory disturbance. One patient presented with persistent vegetative state (apallic syndrome).Seventeen patients did not survive. Twelve of them (70.6%) died of cardiac causes such as reinfarction (3 patients) and pump failure (9 patients) leading to therapy-resistant cardiogenic shock.[68]

Similarly, the EMS system in Göteborg, Sweden, treated 3,754 out-of-hospital cardiac arrests between 1980 and 1993. Twenty-two percent were hospitalized alive, and 9 percent (320) lived to be discharged from the hospital. At discharge, 171 patients had normal neurological functioning or slight neurological deficits; sixty-six had moderate neurological deficits; seventy-seven had severe neurological deficits; and six were in a chronic vegetative state. During the first year, sixty-one of the survivors of cardiac arrest died, and an additional forty-six experienced another arrest. At the end of the first year, 263 survivors were left, and among these, data were available for 212. One hundred fifty-six had normal neurological functioning or slight neurological deficits; eighteen had moderate neurological deficits; thirty-six had severe neurological deficits; and two were in a chronic vegetative state. Only a few survivors were alive after five years, and most had died within ten years of the date of discharge.

A U.S. study shows comparable results. In Birmingham, Alabama, sixty-three children suffered an out-of-hospital cardiopulmonary arrest between 1988 and 1993. Eighteen children were admitted to the intensive-care unit, and six were discharged from the hospital. Five of the survivors had severe neurological deficits, while one had no impairment.

At follow-up, two children had died (one month and seven months after discharge), three were in a permanent vegetative condition, and one appeared normal.[69]

These studies provide startling and dramatic findings. Survival rates hide the Russian roulette aspect of resuscitative efforts. The term "survival rate" highlights lifesaving while it glosses over the possibility— indeed, the likelihood—that these same interventions create neurologically impairment.[70] Because different vital organs can be restored after varying time spans, hearts and lungs will inevitably be restored while brains will not. With CPR, we save lives, but we produce people with a range of disabilities. The two outcomes are inevitably intertwined. Only one of them, however, is used to evaluate resuscitation. Even if we focus on the most promoted side of resuscitative efforts—the 1–3 percent of all people discharged alive—we still do not know much about the meaning of a resuscitative event in the life course of survivors. We do not know how these people incorporate their confrontation with mortality in their biographies, how they interpret their "near-death" experience, how they adjust to "minimal brain damage." Survivors in the Swedish study complained of more "social problems" than they had had before the cardiac arrest.[71] These self-reported measures remain too general to provide much insight. Even less is known about any long-term consequences of resuscitative interventions. The possibility of neurological disabilities is, of course, not a sufficient reason to eliminate resuscitation, but the absence of ethical, medical, and social complications in evaluation research is highly problematic.

More than survival rates, the lives people live after survival— in terms of both length and quality—should be the ultimate criterion for evaluating lifesaving techniques. This issue, however, seems to fall beyond the realm of emergency medicine. The patient admitted to the hospital enters the jurisdiction of neurology and intensive care and is out of the emergency system. As in the past, the resuscitation community's solution to these difficult questions is hoping that the problems will resolve themselves with better techniques. But this reasoning is flawed. If better techniques can save more patients, even more people will be left in a permanent vegetative state.

Still, the next frontier in resuscitation research is brain resuscitation— cardiopulmonary cerebral resuscitation, or CPCR. Since the early seventies, Peter Safar's Pittsburgh center and other research groups have been searching for a means of resuscitating the brain. Their goal is to widen the "window of opportunity" for full recovery after cardiac arrest lasting from five to ten minutes. Until now these research initiatives have not been translated into an easy CPCR protocol: "Reasons for the lack of a cerebral resuscitation breakthrough thus far include the multifactorial complexity of the cerebral postresuscitation syndrome, the unreliability (until recently) of laboratory models, inadequate funding of reliable outcome models, and the limitations of clinical trials."[72] Safar's research group has also been promoting "ultra-advanced life support" to replace CPR, a mechanical and surgical updating of open-chest cardiac massage. These authors seriously suggest that rescuers in the field open veins and arteries and pump blood with an external device such as an oxygenator or a plunger inserted through the ribs.[73] In addition, several researchers have been proposing updated forms of CPR. Noting that coronary perfusion with CPR rarely exceeds more than 30 percent of normal blood output, researchers have proposed a new device that compresses and decompresses the abdomen and chest, or have revisited Claude Beck's idea of open-chest cardiac massage in the field.[74]

While formulating their arguments for new and improved resuscitation techniques, these researchers admit that CPR, with its current survival rates, is unsatisfactory. In 1997, for example, Max Harry Weil and Wanchun Tang published "Cardiopulmonary Resuscitation: A Promise as Yet Largely Unfulfilled," in which they pointed out that after thirty-five years, "the outcome of CPR intervention after 'sudden death' is nevertheless very disappointing." They also state that "the ordering of priorities [in CPR protocols] is based on consensus rather than objective experimental or clinical evidence of improved outcome"[75] and that the resuscitation field has too quickly assumed that the research phase of CPR is finished. Yet even these few medical researchers who admit the limits of CPR do not question the resuscitation project but pave the way for even more medically advanced additions to the current system.

Number-to-Number Inflation

How many people would survive if all emergency medical systems in the United States approached the hypothesized maximum survival rate of 20% that occurs in mature EMS systems? If an estimated 3% survival rate is applied to the presumed annual 400,000 cardiac arrests, approximately 12,000 people per year now survive out-of-hospital cardiac arrest. A 20% survival rate for this population of nontraumatic cardiac arrest patients would yield 80,000 survivors, or an additional 68,000 people. The American Heart Association estimates that nationwide implementation of all life-saving emergency cardiac care mechanisms in each community may save between 100,000 and 200,000 people in the United States.[76]

What do we make of these numbers published by the leading resuscitation researchers? Would we not want to believe these exaggerated numbers and save the equivalent of the population of a midsize town every year? What does an optimal survival rate of 20 percent or 30 percent mean? Imagine a big piece of white paper on which you spill a small drop of black ink. If the white surface represents the number of times that someone engages in CPR, and the black dot represents people who survive, you can see that choices for calculating a survival rate are the first strategic decisions of resuscitation researchers. A survival rate of 1–3 percent also implies a mortality rate of more than 97 percent, and instead of a survival rate, we could evaluate the outcome of resuscitation in terms of mortality rates. But the resuscitation research community decided to focus on the blot instead of the vast white background. Unfortunately, the dot is not prominent enough yet. Resuscitation researchers thus cut about 80 percent off the sheet because the cases lack a good chance of survival. Only patients whose sudden death had cardiac origins and was witnessed, and whom the paramedics found in ventricular fibrillation or ventricular tachycardia, are left on the small scrap of paper. Then, to accentuate the survivors even more, resuscitation researchers take a black pencil and color over the grey values of neurological functioning while, with an eraser, they make the most severely impaired patients disappear into the white background. Finally, they frame their tinkering with a generalization from the best communities. This is the craftwork that produces "the hypothesized maximum survival rate of 20% that occurs in mature EMS systems."

Not surprisingly, the statistical juggling and touched-up survival rates are hidden from the public.[77] Few people have the time and resources to reconstruct these measurements. Because the goal of CPR courses is to have people engage in CPR, survival rates are rarely mentioned during training sessions. I interviewed several CPR and ACLS instructors and ED personnel and found that their estimates of the survival rate varied tremendously, from nearly zero to 80 percent.[78] If the professional rescuers and instructors cannot recognize survival rates, they cannot provide the people they train with the information. The public therefore relies on "real-life" television shows for its knowledge and expectations about CPR. In 1996, researchers analyzed the portrayal of resuscitation on three popular TV shows: *ER, Chicago Hope,* and *Rescue 911.*[79] These survival rates were unrealistically high: immediate survival on TV was an absurd 75 percent, and long-term survival was 67 percent. In addition, most televised cardiac arrests were due to trauma; victims were mostly children, teenagers, and young adults (the average age in Seattle for cardiac arrest was 65 years; in Sweden, it was 67 years); and the shows focused on miraculous recoveries. This misrepresentation distorts expectations for end-of-life decision making. Not surprisingly, physicians in the media,[80] and the television producers themselves,[81] defended this unrealistically positive depiction because it might encourage people to learn and apply CPR.

What happens when people learn about survival rates? In the aftermath of the Patient Self-Determination Act, researchers interviewed a number of elderly patients about their preferences.[82] Previous studies had shown that most elderly patients opted for CPR, but this project asked elderly nursing-home residents first about their preferences, then informed them about the probability of survival to discharge (which was put optimistically between 10% and 17%). Researchers then asked these nursing-home residents again whether they would want to be resuscitated. Before the additional information was given, 41 percent of the 287 respondents opted for CPR. After learning about the survival rate, only 22 percent chose CPR. The researchers concluded, "Discussions among the patient, a clinician, and potential surrogate decision makers yield the most valid advance directives. These discussions should include prognostic information. Patients readily understand this information which influences their preferences regarding CPR. Most older patients do not want CPR once they understand the probability of survival."[83] Several other studies have shown that patients often overestimate their likelihood of survival after CPR, and this misinformation may lead them to opt for resuscitation in hypothetical situations in which survival is extremely unlikely.[84]

THE ECONOMIC COST OF SAVING LIVES

In an age of health-care–cost control, health economists have looked at the monetary cost of attempting to cheat death. For example, a 1996 study in Allentown, Pennsylvania, found a cost of $200 if a physician declared a patient dead on arrival in the ED without continuing resuscitative efforts. Resuscitation in the ED of a patient who does not survive costs an average of $4,150.[85] Children usually received more care regardless of their clinical viability, and their costs were therefore higher. In an Alabama study of sixty-three children with out-of-hospital cardiopulmonary arrest, the average cost for the fifty-seven children who did not survive was $10,667. For those who were discharged, the average cost was $100,000.[86] A model describing the CPR process as a series of decision points estimates a cost per surviving patient at $117,000 if the rate of survival to discharge is 10 percent; $248,000 if the rate is 1 percent; and $544,000 if the rate is 0.2 percent.[87] These numbers, however, still underestimate the real cost of CPR because they do not include the fixed capital cost of running an emergency system—CPR training, equipment, personnel time, and organizational costs. One study based on a community hospital's CPR expenditures estimated the cost of CPR and hospital care at $60,327 for each survivor and the total cost of operating the CPR infrastructure during a twenty-one–month period at $2,352,771.[88] Including all these factors using estimates derived from a collaborative international study, researchers calculated that the cost of CPR per six-month survivor would be $406,605 in 1995 dollars, with a range of $344,314 to $966,759 and $225,892 per quality-adjusted life year (the range was $191,286 to $536,088).[89]

How much money is justifiable to save a human life? The answer to this question becomes ethically muddled in a health-care system in which more than forty million people lack the most basic health care because they are uninsured, underinsured, or precariously insured, and where an estimated $988.5 billion, or 14 percent of the 1995 U.S. GDP, was spent on health care.[90] Still, we can put the cost of CPR in perspective by using other financial indicators. Researchers have calculated the cost of CPR per quality-adjusted life year to be $61,000 and have compared this estimate with the cost per quality-adjusted life year of treating low–birth-weight newborns in an ICU ($8,000), 40-year-old hypertensive males with antihypertensive agents ($16,500), and symptomatic single-vessel angina patients with coronary-bypass graft surgery ($64,000).[91] Or, to put the cost of CPR in a different perspective: in 1995, the federal government established the poverty line at $15,569 for a family of four; the median family income in 1995 was $40,611.[92]

Several analysts have cautiously suggested that universal CPR is futile because the financial cost does not outweigh the benefit of the few lives saved. As one physician explained to me, "If you look at medical resources, you kind of have to start drawing a line. For me to resuscitate that person, I can spend about $5,000 or more in ten minutes. And if you look at that amount of money being expended per person who has an incredibly small chance of ever returning to a functional state once again, you start to realize it is probably not the best thing to do." Ethicists and researchers agree when they state that certain groups of patients (particularly those who do not respond to resuscitative care in the field) should not be resuscitated in the ED because they usurp a disproportionate amount of "scarce" health-care dollars.[93] In the Allentown study, for example, researchers calculated that the health-care savings would have been $72,500 per year if patients were declared dead on arrival instead of given unsuccessful reviving attempts in the ED. National savings were estimated at $14 million.[94]

The widespread use of resuscitation thus reflects a choice of priorities in health care. The emergency medical system indicates a preoccupation with heroic interventions to save a few lives. With resuscitation's marginal success, one wonders whether the resources put into the emergency medical system could not be better invested in the prevention of cardiac arrest. First-line health-care workers are aware of this tension. As one nurse explained:

> My biggest thing right now is worry about somebody who comes in with chest pain and make sure to get them to were they need to be going. So if they have a good outcome, they don't have a cardiac arrest. They get the medicine they are supposed to get. The cardiologist comes in, and they get to cardiac rehab. To me, that is more important and a higher priority than resuscitations. We're supposed to do them and do them well, but they have a low yield. There is a bigger yield on preventing a resuscitation and taking care of the cardiac patient that is alive and breathing.

Extensive CPR programs to save human lives also stand in sharp contrast to the withdrawal of resources in programs to support education, medical care, and rehabilitation of people living with disabilities.[95]

UNIVERSAL LIFESAVING

Since CPR emerged as the most promising resuscitation technique, its promoters have been following an aggressive expansionist and universalist strategy. The principle underlying the emergency medical system for the past decades has been that, with more technology, more people trained in CPR, more autonomy for paramedics, and more defibrillators, more lives will eventually be saved. So far, however, no studies have conclusively shown that lifesaving will increase. Yet any sign that the universalist strategy might not fulfill its promise is redefined as an indication that the community in question has not invested enough resources. A dip in survival rates becomes a rationale for tightening the four links in the "chain of survival" while the structurally flawed principles behind the emergency medical system remain unquestioned. More resources also mean that resuscitative efforts will be used unsuccessfully and, in turn, will depress survival rates and renew the call for more resources. This vicious circle is built into the emergency system. Emergency researchers seem to agree that universal resuscitation—in the sense of reversing all sudden deaths—is actually a misnomer. It would be more appropriate to redefine resuscitation as "defibrillation first-aid" because hearts in ventricular fibrillation seem to have the best chance for survival. Still, CPR, defibrillation, and the emergency medical system are sold to the public as the key to saving all human lives.

The strategy for universal CPR rests partly on deception and carries serious risks. In absolute numbers, it is possible that more lives are saved with the current emergency system than without the emergency infrastructure, but the relative number of lives saved remains disappointingly low. In addition, despite massive investment, an unknown number of patients live with moderate and severe neurological deficits or in permanent vegetative states. These consequences of the universalist strategy could return to haunt emergency medical system providers because the dominant interpretation of survival rates could easily be turned upside down in a number of ways. If with the current infrastructure survival rates remain low, why invest more resources? Why not accept that sudden death is final? With all the problems regarding survival rates—one could basically justify any proportion between zero and 49 percent as accurate[96]—any indication of CPR's "success" is suspicious. As one observer noted, the pressure for financial accountability for universal CPR is also mounting: "Without further demonstration of the value of EMS systems for sustaining the health of our population, cardiac resuscitation programs are likely to be reduced in the face of increasing local government financial distress."[97] Finally, because the universalist strategy depends on full participation, the fear of creating a negative self-fulfilling prophecy is never far away. If it were widely known that with all the resources in place, the survival rate for CPR and the emergency medical system is still as low as 1 to 3 percent for all attempted resuscitation efforts in major cities, and that the victim may well be only partly resuscitated, many people might not bother learning CPR. They might choose not to intervene, or the emergency medial system might be scaled back.

Until now these profound critiques of low survival rates and permanent vegetative conditions have not generated a critical public discussion about the universal application of CPR. Resuscitative efforts are safeguarded because lifesaving is highly regarded. This indirect effect of the universalist strategy is a consequence of public participation. Once the American Heart Association and the American National Red Cross threw their organizational weight behind CPR and invested in national education campaigns, they implied that the postponement of death was everyone's responsibility. Every American could and should participate in attempts to reverse sudden death. Lifesaving thus became a conditioned reflex; part of the popular fascination of "real-life" TV and movies. Because of the concerted activities of emergency organizations, the popular press, and, eventually, juries in courts of law, CPR and defibrillation became the legal standard of care for sudden cardiac arrest outside the hospital.[98]

Resuscitation techniques have changed Americans' understanding about the end of life and, in turn, Americans have given a new meaning to the concept of resuscitation. In the process of making CPR universal the tasks and division of labor between police officers, fire fighters, paramedics, and EMTs shifted and emergency medicine arose as a medical subdiscipline. Laws about transporting dead bodies, the standard of care in sudden death, and traffic congestion in cities were linked to a sprawling invisible emergency network that aims to connect every heart to the most advanced care possible in EDs. Resuscitation beliefs and infrastructure lie at the core of the contemporary gap between the expectation that lives will be saved and the actual outcome of resuscitative efforts. It does not matter how many lives are actually saved with CPR as long as there is hope that simple chest compressions and blowing air into someone's mouth might be effective. The small possibility, supported with carefully constructed survival rates and favorable media portrayals, is still more attractive than accepting the alternative, the finality of sudden death. CPR's advocates have focused on the technical aspect of the technique and on the moral obligation of using it whenever doubt about life occurs. CPR is presented as a second chance and, for now, the millions of Americans who have learned CPR seem to be willing to take that chance. But in the end, most people nevertheless die. In the ethnographic chapters, I explore how in EDs, unrealistic expectations about lifesaving meet the reality of sudden death.

4   Lifesaving in Action

MARGARET MOUTON,[1] a 64-year-old African-American woman, had recently lost her husband in a traffic accident. She was devastated. Her husband would have retired in a few months. Her stepdaughters worried about the difficult grieving process. They took turns staying with her. The morning of October 23, Margaret smiled while gazing out the window, and her oldest stepdaughter caught the smile, and then left for an errand, thinking, "It will be all right. Mom will work through it."

Shivering, George Daniels closed the door behind him one early morning in March. If he hurried, he could jog to the third bridge over the river before going to his mechanic's job at the other end of town. While warming up, he thought about "his boys." Although George and his wife did not have children, he was an enthusiastic 55-year-old baseball coach in the Irish–American little league.

Anna Phillips and Maria Duncan, two sisters of Dutch ancestry, both great-grandmothers, watched a popular TV sitcom in the early afternoon in their trailer. Anna commented that the weather was rather chilly on this Indian summer day. Anna also felt pain in her chest. This was not good, but she did not say anything to her sister. She waited, expecting it to pass. She did not want to go to the hospital. She blamed the taco she had eaten the previous evening and reminded herself to take an antacid at the next commercial break.

The moment that Anna slumped forward in her chair, George hit the pavement in a painful grimace, grasping for his chest, and Margaret was found lying on the living-room floor by her stepdaughter is crucial. It threatens multiple social identities. All three people were embedded in communities that defined them through relationships with family, friends, hobbies, and jobs. Suddenly, however, their failing hearts and lapsed breathing jeopardized these connections. These people were not dead, but if the cardiac arrest could not be reversed soon, they probably would die.

The reactions of those who witness sudden collapse provides insight about the way American people deal with the unexpected interruption of life. At this penultimate moment, what matters most? Seeing someone on the border between life and death, how do people react to the possibility of impending death?

Cardiopulmonary Resuscitation

When she came home, Margaret's stepdaughter Susan found her step-mother lying on the floor. Panicked, Susan phoned 911. The operator directed her in CPR while he sent an ambulance.[2] In her trailer, Anna's sister summoned help from a neighbor, who in turn called 911. No first responder started CPR on her. At the bridge, George became a victim when a passerby turned him in a face-up position, listened for breathing, felt for a pulse, and yelled to his friend that somebody should call an ambulance. He then hyperextended George's neck and blew air into the open mouth while closing the nose with his hand. With resistance of the lungs and rising of the chest, he concluded that air was going into the lungs. Then he felt for the notch in the middle of the chest (the xiphoid complex), measured two fingers more to the left, and gave fifteen deep compressions with his arms straight and the heel of his hands on George's chest. He followed this protocol with two rescuing breaths, fifteen compressions, two rescuing breaths, and so forth in a steady pattern.

The onset of a resuscitative effort is a culturally significant moment: if we choose to resuscitate, we intend to avoid death. Dying, in contrast, demands a passive attitude. It means letting go and facing the inevitable. But CPR fits a form of human instrumental rationality. The chest compressions and rescue breaths become a means to an end: the certainty of death at the end of a life becomes a probability. The threat of death becomes the promise of a continued life. The choice for CPR is thus a choice for action, for intervention, and for control; ultimately, it is an attempt at immortality in light of pending death.

A paramedic told me that he chose his profession because as a first responder he had once used CPR. "I felt lucky I knew CPR," he explained, "because I could do something." "Doing something" helps establish an atmosphere that feels both inevitable and inviolate. The rhythmic chest compressions and rescue breaths have a soothing effect. If we just do CPR right, everything will be fine. CPR restores a sense of order when the chaos of death looms, and in this sense the resuscitative effort is a ritual. It provides meaning in the face of impending sudden death. As the anthropologist Robbie Davis-Floyd observed: "To perform a series of rituals is to feel oneself locking onto a set of cosmic gears which will safely and inevitably crank the individual right on through the perceived danger to safety on the other side."[3] When the danger is sudden death, the rhythmic motions of CPR provide a sense of comfort.

The cardiac arrest left Margaret in a liminal state, between death and life. In our culture, life and death form a binary opposition. We are either dead or alive. The liminal state is temporary. It will refold soon into one category or the other. Whether Margaret will remain a stepmother, widow, retired teacher, and hospital volunteer, or whether she instead will become a deceased person, depends upon the success of the resuscitation. Those identities, which constituted Margaret as a social being in a community, do matter during the reviving attempt. When Margaret's stepdaughter fought for her stepmother's life, she had a strong emotional kinship connection guiding her efforts. The CPR motions may be automatic, almost obliterating conscious decision making, but Susan knew from all the years of living with her stepmom that her interventions were what Margaret would want. Susan also had an important personal stake in reviving. Whatever the outcome of the reviving effort, she would have to live with the emotional and spiritual implications of her decision to resuscitate.

For first responders who know the unconscious victim, the decision to resuscitate is an extension of established conversations and relationships. Yet even if the rescuer and victim are strangers, clues about the victim's social identities might still indicate the appropriateness of the intervention. The wedding ring on George's finger; his jogging outfit; his sex, race, and age remind the rescuer of the multiple identities George holds.[4] The rescuer who assumed that he shared important values with George will in turn justify a decision to intervene. The rescuer also had a personal stake in engaging in the reviving effort: perhaps he hoped that someone would revive him if he were to collapse. When relatives, friends, or strangers attempt to revive, they reflect values of reciprocity, community, and altruism, and they acknowledge a personal stake in their intervention.

Once such a connection is established, efforts to manage the uncertainty between life and death become standard, memorized resuscitation protocols. The medical algorithms do not draw attention to George's life accomplishments, his skills as a mechanic, or his relationship with his friends and relatives. Instead, they emphasize the failure of his body. His lungs "stopped functioning" and his heart "gave out." Because of the medical interventions that frame the actions, the signs of impending death are associated with weakness, decay, deterioration, and failure.

They signify a process that should be stopped and reversed. From the beginning, resuscitating implies turning away from death. Death hovers over the event, but as the wrong outcome, the state to be avoided.

The two main components of CPR, mouth-to-mouth ventilation and chest compressions, reflect a Western approach to life and death. Instead of "re-animating" (bringing back the *anima*, or soul), "re-suscitating" (to raise or revive) consists of restoring somebody's heart and lungs. As Margaret Lock has pointed out, in Japan, where the body and mind are believed to be mutually connected, "an individual cannot be declared dead until the embodied spirit had ceased to function."[5] For many other cultures, vitality is a matter of balancing energy forces. The Chinese *yin* and *yang* and the flow and constitution of *chi* (vital energy) are one example.[6] Our focus on the heart and lungs to signify death perpetuates a profound mind–body split. During CPR, a person is "alive" when he or she is breathing unassisted and has a heartbeat, regardless of the neurological functioning. With the heart and lungs as indicators of death, CPR is behind the times. Legally (especially in light of organ procurement)[7] someone is dead once brain activity stops, even if a pulse or breathing is observable.

CPR is unusual in the way it brings strangers into intimate contact. Its actions combine the intimate and the violent. First the rescuer "kisses" the unconscious person, then "hits" the person hard. We love life, hate death, love life, hate death in a perpetual rhythm. Mouth-to-mouth ventilation remains an unarousing sexual act, while chest compressions are deliberate beneficial and measured blows. Putting one's lips on a dying stranger's lips and violently pounding his or her chest would violate the "territories of the self"[8] if these actions were not part of standard resuscitative protocols. Before someone can administer these lifesaving motions, the rescuer must perform a mini-assessment: checking for breathing, making sure that the airway is unobstructed, and feeling for a pulse. Only when the airway is established and pulse and breathing remain absent should CPR be initiated. Consent for these procedures is assumed when a person is unconscious. First responders pay attention to the number of compressions and rescue breaths, the positions of their hands, and the airtight seal around the mouth and nose. They monitor the rising of the chest, pace their rescue breaths with a helpful mnemonic, and try to give smooth, rhythmic, and uninterrupted compressions. These ritualistic precautions affirm that a resuscitative effort is a dispassionate, nonviolent encounter.

But ritualistic precautions do not render the rescuer invincible. According to the Basic Life Support instructor's manual,[9] trainees usually raise two sets of concerns: infectious diseases and legal liability. The socially constructed stigma attached to HIV infection turns every contact, intimate or not, between strangers suspicious. Nurse Jennifer Cohen noted, "If a stranger drops on the street, you always have that option to walk by, . . . and I have to admit to a lot of apprehension to [engage in CPR] if somebody drops in the mall. I don't know what I'm dealing with, and I'm not sure I'm going to give mouth-to-mouth resuscitation to this person who may have AIDS or resistant tuberculosis. I think I'm going to be the one who goes to dial 911." A respiratory therapist added, "Nowadays, with AIDS in the community, you have people who are thinking twice about just trying [to resuscitate]. Even myself: in the past, I would not have thought anything about it, but now I hesitate. Do I want to do this?"

One study showed that in 1993, 80 percent of interviewed nurses declined to perform mouth-to-mouth ventilation because of the fear of acquiring infectious diseases.[10] Michael Perry described how he performed bystander CPR on an accident victim who later tested HIV-positive.[11] Although Perry wore gloves, they ripped, and he came in contact with the victim's blood. Reflecting on this experience, Perry noted, "In the past, the average person on the street wouldn't hesitate to help an accident victim. Now fears, both founded and unfounded, threaten to quell this spirit. The decision to give care has been transformed from a snap decision to a daunting ethical dilemma." [12] The "founded and unfounded" fears about infection clash with the moral values of rendering aid to people in an emergency. The solution to these fears is to dilute the risks of infection in CPR-training sessions—"In the absence of evidence of risk for infectious diseases, including AIDS, the lifesaving potential of CPR should continue to be vigorously emphasized, and energetic efforts in support of broadscale CPR training should be continued"[13]—and to rely on "HIV-resistant" face shields and masks. These aids are controversial, however, because people might not want to engage in CPR when the masks are unavailable. A rescuer also needs two hands to handle the mask and maintain an open airway, and therefore the masks are recommended only for CPR performed by two rescuers.

With malpractice litigation permeating every aspect of medicine, many people also express legal concerns about rendering first-aid. According to U.S. common law, "A person making a well-intentioned but incompetent attempt to rescue another is held legally liable, whereas failure to act may not produce legal consequences."[14] This situation, in which moral principles of beneficence are pitched against common-law principles, gave rise to the Good Samaritan immunity statutes. These vary from state to state, but all provide immunity from legal liability if a rescuer's actions rest upon "a good-faith belief that the possible benefits of the attempt outweigh the risk from the rescuer's incompetence."[15] Minnesota and Vermont have gone even further, requiring people to offer emergency assistance. Even so, most of these Good Samaritan provisions and similar professional immunity laws have not been tested in court and depend themselves on "good faith." An EMT handbook concluded that "Although the immunity laws may provide some protection, it is clear that much better protection is provided by rendering top-quality emergency medical care."[16]

The fear of litigation and infection has not eroded people's willingness to engage in resuscitation efforts to the extent that health officials view non-engagement as a significant social problem. Yet, like organ procurement, blood donation, and surrogate motherhood, CPR reveals a pattern of conflicting values resolved in favor of a religiously derived tradition of altruism and self-sacrifice to save others. In contrast with organ donation and surrogate motherhood, however, CPR does not require major or complicated sacrifices. Anyone with two arms and a healthy pair of lungs can provide lifesaving actions. CPR also eases the pain of survivor guilt. A rescuer performing CPR will avoid feeling guilty about helplessly watching someone die.

Therefore, in many ways, resuscitative efforts outside the hospital take place in a communal context. These interventions require a profound level of interpersonal solidarity, based on a belief that every human being would want to live and be rescued by others. CPR relies on the collaboration between strangers to engage in reviving efforts regardless of age, race, sex, sexual orientation, physical and mental abilities, political preferences, or other differences.[17] The American Heart Association and Red Cross have encouraged potential rescuers to forget about infection and liability. We necessarily have all become implicated in this modernist project of achieving immortality by instrumental means. The emergency medical system functions only if most people are willing to engage in lifesaving and, in turn, want to be saved. The lifesaving technology transfers the power of life and death to everyone.[18] This diffusion of power requires constant surveillance of everyone by everyone. The protocols, however, point to the insufficiency of these lifesaving interventions: they imply that to be successful, resuscitation requires specialized professional care. The rationale of a resuscitative effort is to enable the administration of more advanced care such as electric defibrillation and intravenous drug therapies. Therefore, the first step of a protocol is to alert the emergency medical system. The message is clear: you cannot do it alone; professionals need to come and help you out.

When the paramedics arrive, an important shift occurs. The lifesaving actions embedded in community ties, reciprocity, and altruism now become professional and medical. The resuscitative effort becomes more invasive, and the rites to reverse the dying process become more elaborate. These more advanced reviving interventions come at a great cost: the needs of relatives and friends who face loss through the impending death are subservient to the concerns of the medical profession. The more humane aspects of resuscitation give way to increasing biomedical lifesaving power.

PARAMEDICS

When the ambulance stopped at Margaret's suburban house, John Lavinger, a paramedic, jumped out, opened the back door, and grabbed a portable defibrillator and a big orange box filled with medications. His colleague, Bob Winchester, radioed the time of arrival to the 911 station and followed with a stretcher and an oxygen tank. They entered the house and walked into the living room. While John asked Margaret's stepdaughter Susan what had happened, he felt for Margaret's carotid and radial pulses. He quickly cut through her pajamas and connected the three leads of the portable heart monitor, which provided information about the electrical activity of the heart. In the meantime, he asked about his patient's age, previous medical history, specific allergies to drugs, and the medication she was taking. He then continued the heart compressions that Susan had begun. Bob connected an air mask with reservoir to the oxygen tank, intubated his patient by putting an airway tube into her throat, and put the mask on her face. He forced the oxygen into her lungs by squeezing the reservoir. Air moved through the endotracheal tube. The paramedics glanced at the rhythm on the portable defibrillator. They looked at each other, and John said, "Let's get her out of here." They turned their patient on her side and slid her onto a backboard. They carefully lifted the backboard onto a stretcher.

Bob steered the stretcher while John continued chest compressions and ventilations. John asked Susan whether she had a preference for a particular hospital, then they left with sirens wailing. Similar scenarios were followed for Anna and George. George was particularly lucky because he collapsed close to the ambulance station, and paramedics arrived instantly after the call.

With the arrival of the paramedics, Anna, George, and Margaret entered a patient–health-care provider relationship. Whereas the term "victim" still connotes someone trapped in an uncontrollable situation, the term "patient" refers to a controlled, passive party excused from everyday obligations and charged with getting better.[19] The patient–paramedic relationship presumes a professional distance, announced by the ambulance's wailing siren, the clean white or neutral blue uniform, the stethoscope, the radio attached to the shoulder, and medical paraphernalia hanging off the belt.

Paramedics do not engage in the very intimate mouth-to-mouth ventilation and often do not perform chest compressions. They rely on mechanical aids. Instead of hyperextending the person's neck, they intubate by placing a tube in the trachea. Instead of mouth-to-mouth ventilation, they slide an oxygen mask over the patient's face, and push a bag to direct 100 percent oxygen into the lungs. In some emergency systems, the paramedics also locate the patient under "the thumper," a device that compresses the chest at set intervals. The clinical rationale behind the mechanized interventions is that mechanical means are more reliable and powerful, and therefore have more reviving potential than manual substitutes. But mechanization also implies that CPR performed by relatives or first responders is insufficient and that the fight to prevent death is an advanced medical task. Indeed, one of the key characteristics of being a professional is to have official jurisdiction over some area of social life.[20]

The official reason behind stripping Margaret of her pajamas is easy access to the chest, to fasten the defibrillator electrodes and check the pulse points in the groin. Clothes, however, are also markers of individuality. Nuns, Marine basic trainees, and prisoners leave their clothes behind when they enter the convent, training camp, or prison. In these settings, removing clothes during a resuscitative effort means submitting to uniformity. It also indicates that the person is no longer autonomous but dependent, in this case, on medical professionals.[21] The rules safeguarding the autonomous self are no match for the task of saving a human life. Under the mandate of working as fast as possible, paramedics do not care about shame or prudishness. They expose private body parts to the public eye. While the patient's body is invaded, the body boundaries of the paramedics are enclosed and protected by machines, face masks, and a double pair of latex gloves. CPR requires intensive human contact, but the paramedics create protective barriers between themselves and their patients. The patient is treated as a potentially infectious body from whom the medical representatives need to be protected. Once these precautions are in place, the paramedic's license to act increases. The precautions acknowledge the vulnerability and mortality of the professional rescuer.[22]

Because they are professionals paid to rescue people, paramedics do not act out of altruism, friendship, family ties, or hope for reciprocity. The altruistic principles are at the center of their professional credo, usually under a variation of the Hippocratic oath, but those principles are subordinate to the rule of self-protection. Emergency personnel are prohibited from entering an accident scene if their own safety cannot be guaranteed. They first need to "secure the scene," even if it means that important time is lost.

Sooner or later, novice paramedics and physicians learn that another ethical principle is more important than the Hippocratic oath. Health-care providers refer to it as "CYA" (cover your ass[ets]). When the young physician James Dillard stopped at a car accident and pulled a man out of the car, probably saving the victim's life but creating the possibility of rendering him quadriplegic, his professor lectured him, "Well, you did the right thing medically, of course. But, James, do you know what you put at risk by doing that?" "What was I supposed to do?" I asked. "Drive on," he replied. "There is an army of lawyers out there who would stand in line to get a case like that. If that driver had turned out to be a quadriplegic, you might never have practiced medicine again. You were a very lucky young man."[23] This example underscores the moral and legal dilemmas facing health-care providers. The legal implications of the rescue case could have ruined the young health-care provider both financially and professionally, and, as James regretfully agreed with his professor, that risk did outweigh saving a human life.

Professionalization of lifesaving means that when the paramedics arrive, the relatives, friends, and first responders step aside. Although resuscitating signifies human control over death, it now moves out of the relatives' reach. The lungs and hands of relatives and friends are not only considered too inexperienced to revive effectively, but relatives also are powerless in the decision-making process. They cannot negotiate a partial resuscitative effort, perhaps with only CPR and without drugs or IVs or with limits placed on the revival attempt. They cannot ask for advice to reach an informed decision about whether to resuscitate. They cannot request that paramedics declare their loved one dead. The paramedics have standing orders stipulating that unless very obvious signs of death are present (such as decapitation, massive head trauma, advanced rigor mortis, or a body consumed by fire), they will have to resuscitate and transport the patient to the emergency department.[24] They may assume that consent for all those procedures is given. Even if the patient has an advance directive and the relatives have the document ready, paramedics are legally obligated to continue the resuscitative effort. In most counties, paramedics may not interpret advance directives. Only physicians—who remain in the ED—are allowed to act upon these documents and stop a reviving effort.

The arrival of the paramedics means shifting gears from a rhythmic manual intervention to a highly technological medical procedure. A whole set of social identities becomes temporarily irrelevant for the professional rescuers. It does not matter that Anna was a great-grandmother with a sister, a home, and community ties. What matters is that she mistook chest pain for indigestion and did nothing about it. As patients, Anna, George, and Margaret are redefined as people with a particular physiological condition (nonfunctioning heart and lungs), who are found in certain circumstances, and who have or do not have a medical history that would explain the cardiac failure. As patients, they become a set of narrow medical parameters, such as blood pressure, pulse, EKG reading, and possible reaction to medication. When the paramedics wheel their stretcher into the ambulance, they disregard medically irrelevant identities and, by following the CPR script, attribute a new set of medical identities, centered on cardiac arrest.[25]

The official resuscitation theory allows only four to six minutes of oxygen deprivation before irreversible brain damage occurs. The paramedics take a couple of minutes to reach the patient, and they do not know for sure how long the patient has been without oxygen. But they remember how long their patient was unconscious in their hands, and they also realize that if the patient is going to revive without severe neurological damage, that patient needs to respond quickly to the treatment. A paramedic summarized the importance of time and timing,

"You are fighting time. You don't have a whole lot of time to do it. You'd better be working quickly, because time will be stealing away any chance you have. CPR is a fight for time, and it is time-dependent." Therefore, experienced paramedics often realize that the patient is beyond lifesaving, especially after they read the EKG rhythm and note the lack of response to drugs and medication. For them, death is not a potential threat anymore but an embodied reality. But because of the way the emergency medical system is structured, paramedics have to keep resuscitating. Death has not legally occurred yet. Therefore, the paramedics administer drugs, shock the body, and dutifully note everything they find. Usually, they go through the motions of the protocol without expecting that the promised result—a saved life—will be obtained. Still, even as they perform the obligatory tasks, their actions create a sense of continuity and predictability for bystanders and relatives.

In contrast to the often clumsy and hesitant motions of relatives and first responders, the smoothness of the paramedics' actions sends a powerful message that the professional rescuers are going to be able to reverse the dying process. The use of an automatic defibrillator adds to the drama and the magic of the resuscitative performance. The automatic defibrillator reads the invisible electrical charges in the heart and sends out a beeping warning tone. The paramedics warn the bystanders to stand clear, and the body shocks violently with a charge of up to 360 joules, limbs often flailing in the air. Besides the increased use of technological gadgets, most people associate professional rescuers with almost definite survival. Their assumptions come from popular TV shows in which paramedics achieve unrealistically high survival rates. Thus, when paramedics arrive, bystanders often breathe a sigh of relief. They feel that the danger of death is gone when the professional rescuers quickly assess the patient and wheel their loved one into the ambulance. The brisk, routinized actions of the paramedics create a sense of control over the threatening situation. When the ambulance takes off for the hospital, relatives and first responders hang on to a sliver of hope that things will work out after all.

THE EMERGENCY DEPARTMENT

In the ED, the basic goal of the technology—saving lives fast—remains the same as it was in the field, but the number of actors and instruments increases. While the staff works on the patient, the community aspects that provided meaning to resuscitation interventions become irrelevant. The community—family, friends, bystanders—has no place in the ED until a decision about the patient is made and the effort is over. The medical and nursing staff work through a more complicated resuscitation protocol than CPR. Their protocols are grouped in a set of algorithms that form Advanced Cardiac Life Support (ACLS).

The paramedics notified the ED of their impending arrival with Anna. The nurse who took the call gave the "code blue" warning. The department secretary paged the respiratory therapists, who were working all over the hospital.[26] The nurse who took the call assembled a physician, an emergency technician, and a colleague in the resuscitation room when the ambulance was only three to four minutes away. A second technician waited outside for the ambulance. She opened the ambulance doors and helped to put the stretcher outside. "How is she?" she asked. The paramedic answered: "Asystole." This single term, referring to a flat line of the EKG monitor, encapsulated Anna's condition and defined expectations for likely outcomes. Together the two paramedics wheeled the patient inside while the technician stood on the bar at the bottom and performed chest compressions. In the room, the paramedics lifted the patient from the stretcher onto the bed.

Immediately, an entire team began a variety of tasks on the body. The respiratory therapists took care of the ventilation. They checked the intubation to make sure that the lungs (and not the stomach) were ventilated. They attached their own air mask with reservoir to Anna's face and continued ventilating her with 100 percent oxygen. The technician, standing on a little stool, gave chest compression to stimulate the circulation. Physicians and nurses shared the job of monitoring Anna's condition and administering drugs. They established IV lines to pumps and gave fluids and medications. They checked her temperature and blood pressure and the dilation level of her eyes. If indicated, they would also defibrillate the heart with electrical countershocks. A new task emerged as the team took over: taking notes. Standing centrally, a notetaker wrote down Anna's cardiac rhythm when she entered the resuscitation room and noted the drugs and electric shocks that the paramedics administered.

The resuscitation team consisted further of visitors who popped in and out to perform their specific tasks. Radiologists took a chest X-ray, a phlebotomist took blood for analysis, and a special technician used the twelve-lead EKG machine. Outside the resuscitation room, a secretary tried to retrieve Anna's charts, and a chaplain or a social worker comforted Anna's family and neighbors who had arrived in the ED. The ACLS procedures brought all these professionals together and ordered them as a team. Every one of these people gathered information about Anna's condition and viability and transmitted this information to the notetaker and the physician. After the first rush, the resuscitative effort calmed down. Chest compressions and artificial ventilation continued, and the physician ordered a number of drugs. The effort needed to carry on for at least ten to fifteen minutes to determine whether Anna would react positively to the pharmaceuticals.

The actions and emotions of the emergency personnel create the impression that the threat of death is remote. Even if a patient's body is not showing any signs of viability, it is at the center of a bustling of activity and energy. The moving, talking, touching, pumping, writing, running in and out, and bustling of eight to twenty-five people in a room brightly lit with white neon lights creates a lively atmosphere. Pumps flash lights. Monitors sound alarms. Like surgical teams that unite emotionally,[27] a resuscitative effort has an emotional feel. Jim Atkins, a young physician, explained, "The way the person who is running the code [directs the team] sort of filters through the whole room. If you get someone in there who is inexperienced at it or someone who has never felt comfortable with it, everybody feels uncomfortable." The team's emotion can be uncomfortable or hectic, but rarely is there a sense of impending doom or overwhelming sorrow in the room.

I am often asked how I could handle observing such intense life-and-death dramas, but most resuscitative efforts carry no intensity or drama. Team members are calm, doing their jobs and conversing with each other. Sometimes mistakes happen, or drugs are in short supply, and people yell at each other. But more often there is laughter in the room. In the community where I observed resuscitation, the paramedics and emergency-room staff are friends. While helping each other out, they joke around and exchange stories and invitations to parties. During reviving efforts, it was difficult to sense the sadness and solemnity that we associate with death and dying. The organization of the emergency institution, the actions detailed in protocols, and the routine character of interventions with such low survival rates strengthen the emotional distance between the staff and the dying patient. But this distance is deceiving. It suggests that every contingency is under control. Instead, because time has elapsed, irreversible biological death often has already occurred.

At the center of the staff's attention is the EKG monitor, with its characteristic irregular line and beeping signals. The combination of visual and auditory rhythmic stimuli pace and synchronize the resuscitative effort. Josh Brittan, a technician, expressed this the best: "Actually, when I'm doing compressions and focused on my job, I'm not really aware of who else is around me. Personally, I usually pick a spot on the monitor, and I concentrate. I try to make it cohesive enough between myself and the people doing the breathing. Once you develop a sync, you really aren't aware of everybody else around. I have been aware [of distractions], and I try not to let them change what I'm doing. Because once you get into sync, everything else around you no longer matters." The wiggling line of the EKG monitor also captures the condition of the patient and justifies decisions and actions. The objective knowledge of the machine is more authoritative than the team's subjective knowledge. At the end of a resuscitative effort in which the patient dies, a nurse needs to have an imprint of the EKG rhythm in different leads to document and prove that the patient is indeed officially dead.

In both hospitals where I observed resuscitative attempts, specially trained ACLS nurse administrators took extensive notes about the sequence and administration of the drugs, tubes, EKG rhythms, outcomes, and decisions during the resuscitative effort. These detailed written records serve billing purposes, but more important, the documentation helps to cover the team in malpractice lawsuits. If legal disputes arise, the notes will be used as evidence. Hospital administrators make sure that every step is recorded along the way. In the resuscitation process, the protocols are prominent. According to the American Heart Association (which publishes the ACLS and CPR guidelines), the protocols are intended as guidelines for the physician's decision making, but in reality the protocols play a more directive and evaluative role in the resuscitative attempt. The resuscitation protocols specify dosages and amounts of drugs, the time to start compressions, the rate of ventilation, the percentage of oxygen in the reservoir, the places to look for a pulse, the time to take an X-ray, and so forth. Checking a laminated copy of the protocol, which they carry in their pockets, administrators in the room regularly interfere in the reviving effort. They may remind the physician that according to the ACLS protocols, it is time to give a new dose of epinephrine, or they may explain that the patient cannot be declared legally dead because the protocol is not yet exhausted. For the hospital bureaucracy, creating a complete record becomes a goal in itself.

In the ED, internal vital functions are on display outside the body. George's heart was connected to an EKG monitor, which also registered the pulse in his finger and automatically took his blood pressure. Margaret's veins were connected to intravenous lines with different solutions and drugs. These lines were themselves linked to beeping pumps that regulated the solution's dosages. Margaret's lungs were attached directly through an endotracheal tube to an oxygen reservoir and later to an automatic ventilator. Anna's chest X-rays showed whether her heart was enlarged or her lungs were clouded. A blood sample was analyzed for the oxygen and pH levels. A twelve-lead EKG monitor exposed not only the electrical activity in her heart but also the electrical activity throughout her entire body.

The boundaries of a patient's body are extended through lines and electrodes. Body functions become the province of other people and machines. The result is that Anna's status was uncertain. She could be either biologically alive or dead. Equally uncertain was where she stopped or began. The machines, the pumps, the intravenous lines, and the rhythmic hand movements of the respiratory therapist and the technician became part of her. They took care of her vital functions; to remove these externalized organs[28] was to interrupt her lifeline.

In the ED, medical identities have become the main identifiers of patients.[29] Great-grandmothers and sisters are replaced by lines on a screen, numbers on a piece of paper. But this process of increasing ambiguity between life and death cannot continue forever. Time works against ambiguity. The person in cardiac arrest is like a surfer at the cresting moment of a wave. The surfer is at a pivotal point and either rides the wave or falls into the water.[30] In the ED, the person in cardiac arrest is at the same sort of peak transformational moment: medicine and technology are maximized, and the patient's viability is transformed into the smallest set of indicators. Breathing and circulation are artificially incited with chemicals, manual manipulation, and electricity. Not much more can be done.

Two outcomes are possible. Soon it becomes obvious that even the tightest links between technology and the failing lungs and heart will not suffice to save a life. After ten minutes of a reviving effort, Anna did not regain any signs of life. The physician who left the room to take care of other patients prepared to declare her dead by turning to the team and asking them if they had any suggestions for further resuscitating. When nobody answered her question, the physician looked at the clock and said, "All right then. Let's stop. It's 10:35." The notetaker then recorded the time of death, and the team dispersed.

Margaret was on a roller-coaster. The drugs and other medical interventions were only temporary means to restore life. Margaret had a rhythm defined as reasonable by the ACLS script, but when compressions stopped and the drugs wore off, the rhythm disappeared and the monitor showed a flat line. The intravenous lines ceased running because her circulation was inadequate. Her blood gases remained very low, even after the prescribed high-sodium bicarbonate and higher rates of hyperventilating.[31] She was also pronounced dead.

In an apparently successful resuscitation, in contrast, the medical linkages seem effective at first sight. Hesitatingly, George's body regained a pulse. The heartbeat was palpable first in the groin and later in the neck and the wrists. The attending physician heard definite heartbeats with the stethoscope. The EKG monitor showed a regular, viable rhythm, so that blood pressure could be measured. George's blood pressure, however, remained worrisomely low, barely noticeable. When the results of the blood gases came back from the lab, they told the team that George was not adequately perfused for someone in his condition. The physician decided nevertheless to summon a ventilator from the intensive-care unit, and George was prepared for transfer. While the fluids and EKG screen were carefully monitored, the nurse taking notes stroked the dull end of a pen against the soles of George's feet to examine his reflexes. George did not twitch or move—a bad sign. The respiratory therapist checked with a small flashlight whether his pupils were dilated, open, cloudy, or clear. The eyes reacted sluggishly to the light. The reflexes and state of the pupils indicated problems with George's neurological status.

Whatever the result, the ambiguity between life and death ends with a decision about the patient's status. At that turning point, the resuscitation effort ceases and a life has been either saved or lost. In an abrupt transition, the momentum of the activity is reversed. Whether the patient has died or been stabilized, the tight medical linkages and the medical identities are removed (or at least loosened), and the body resumes its previous social multiplicity. The members of the emergency medical staff pay attention to some of the social cues and community connections that they had disregarded earlier. The body becomes again a part of a social network. Someone will ask, "Do we have a name?" or "Is the family here?" The chaplain or social worker answers these questions.

In contrast with only moments earlier when death seemed far removed, its signs now permeate every corner of the resuscitation room. The team that was previously bustling around has largely left the room, taking with them the laughter, machine noise, and red digital flashing alarms. The white neon light that lit the room now seems too bright. A technician switches it off and, in turn, lights a smaller and softer yellow lamp above the bed. A box with tissues is kept handy to give to crying relatives. While moments before the nurses were inserting IVs and touching the body all over, they now keep a respectable distance from the deceased patient. Even when they wipe away the blood, their touch has a re-found gentle and caring sensitivity. They pity Margaret for dying so young and leaving children behind and envy Anna's relatively quick passing.

In Margaret's case, the shift occurred once the resuscitation team decided that her situation was hopeless. The social worker entered the resuscitation room and mentioned Margaret Mouton's name. Joan Judis, one of the nurses, remembered her from three weeks earlier when her husband died in the same ED. She remarked that Margaret looked different without a wig. Judis recalled that Margaret was upset and had needed something to calm her down. The social worker added that this measure may be necessary for her stepdaughters, as well, because they are very distressed and insist on seeing their stepmother. While these issues were being discussed, and when the physician decided that Margaret was in fact dead, the respiratory therapist took off the oxygen reservoir, threw it in the garbage, and left. The technician stopped compressions and put Margaret's ripped clothes in a plastic bag. Judis switched off the monitor, unplugged the leads, and took off the blood-pressure cuff. She closed the fully dilated eyes, and wiped the blood off Margaret's face. She put Margaret's body in a hospital gown. Then she took a clean sheet and covered Margaret up to the head. She hid the hand with the punctures and bruises of the intravenous connections under the sheet while the other hand remained visible. The empty boxes and wrappings of drugs and solutions were thrown away. The only remaining trace of the medical work was the tube in Margaret's mouth, which the nurse could not take out before the coroner released the body.[32] Except for this tube, Margaret laid peacefully, a sleeping body in an almost empty room. The technician put two chairs in the room. Judis waited until the chaplain arrived with the family members.

Dr. Martine Chau, the physician in charge of Margaret's reviving attempt, walked into the counseling room where the two stepdaughters waited anxiously with the social worker. The social worker, who had run back and forth between the counseling room and the resuscitation room, had already prepared the two women, saying, "It doesn't look very good." Dr. Chau entered, closed the door, sat down, and said, "I have bad news. Mrs. Mouton died." The stepdaughters started crying and fell into each other's arms. The physician explained that their stepmom probably died from a massive cardiac infarction and that very little could have been done when she arrived in the ED. She asked whether they had any questions. Susan wondered whether her stepmother had died in pain. The physician replied that when Margaret entered the ED, she was unconscious and probably could not feel anything anymore. The social worker then asked Dr. Chau whether it would be OK to visit the body. The physician gave her permission. As they left the room, the social worker prepared the women for the way the body would look. He especially mentioned the tube in the throat. In the resuscitation room, Judis encouraged Margaret's stepdaughters to take the hand of their now deceased stepmother and touch it. Susan told about the loss of her father and how her stepmother had grieved. She recalled how that morning she had felt relieved because her stepmom seemed to feel happier. She felt the feet and remarked that they were cold. Her sister remembered how her father used to tell his wife, "If I had known how cold your feet were, I wouldn't have married you." She added, "She wanted to be with Pop."

Margaret's stepdaughters' grieving and their stories restore Margaret to the social network. She is now a dead person, not an ambiguous body machine reduced to basic medical parameters. Her identities are now partly and gradually reinvoked and redefined to match her new condition of a deceased person. The coroner's examination of the body,[33] the questions about their choice of funeral home, and the requests for organ donation confirm the firmness and inevitability of this new identity. For the first time since Margaret and Anna fell down, their relatives are encouraged to think of death as a reality.

George, who precariously survived the resuscitative effort, also assumed a new identity. The reviving attempt marked the beginning of his status as a neurology and cardiac patient. A CT scan, MRI, and other tests in the intensive-care unit had detected a seriously abnormal cardiac rhythm, and the heart surgeon would have liked to implant an internal pacemaker but hesitated because George remained in a comatose condi-

tion. If the surgery went forward, George would have faced a lengthy recovery process and a strict rehabilitation regimen. The cardiac arrest also
required a redefinition of his personal biography. In the unlikely event
that George recovered, he would need to fit his new identity of a chronic
heart patient with other identities.[34] George would need to reconsider
how much time to spend in his old job, how active to be as a sports coach,
and whether he wanted to follow the dietary changes his doctor suggested. The poet Audre Lorde[35] described the biographical work[36]
prompted by an increased awareness of mortality, "There were different
questions about time that I would have to start asking myself. Not, for
how long do I stand at the window and watch the dawn coming up over
Brooklyn, but rather, how many more new people do I admit so openly
into my life? I needed to examine and pursue the implications of that
question. It meant plumbing the depths and possibilities of relating with
the people already in my life, deepening and exploring them."

At the end of the reviving attempt, the strong message is that death
becomes real only after a physician has united the person with the new
identity of deceased. A biological death needs to be joined with a socially defined death. The physician as ultimate decision maker finalizes
that sudden death is a medical condition that can be treated like any
other disease or illness. This medicalization is reinforced to the outside
world when the physician officially communicates the outcome of the
reviving effort to the relatives and friends. Like the priest in earlier
times, the physician has become the authoritative mediator between
life and death. The death that physicians mediate, however, is a biological death, and, strictly speaking, the resuscitation work ends when
relatives are informed of the death of their loved one. The social ramifications of grieving and coming to terms with passing on are left to
medical adjuncts: chaplains, social workers, and nurses. Dealing with
grieving relatives has a residual quality in hospitals. It depends on the
availability and willingness of staff to engage in the low-valued "caring" instead of the highly valued "curing."

Ritual, Medicalization, and Community

Contradictions abound in resuscitative efforts: people who value indi-
vidualism more than anything else engage in potentially life-threatening altruistic acts. After three decades of patient rights, second opinions,
and health-care–provider choices, people rely submissively and uncrit-

ically on the words of doctors to reveal and accept the final reality of death. In the reviving process, people are reduced to mere bodies, and their dignity is repeatedly violated. During the resuscitative effort, a sharp division exists between what the sociologist Erving Goffman called "frontstage" and "backstage" activities.[37] The frontstage encompasses emotional and spiritual connections. At the backstage, such death-related emotions are absent. A temporal gap also separates biological and legal definitions of death. The most glaring contradiction, however, appears under the guise of reviving. People usually die during resuscitative efforts, and although most people consider this outcome negative, no one regards low survival rates as a sufficient reason to discontinue current protocols.

For outsiders, resuscitative attempts are unlikely to make sense. They seem futile, at best a procedure to trick gullible minds into accepting sudden death. For the bystanders who participate in CPR or the people who are the most affected by sudden death, however, resuscitative efforts might seem the best way currently available to die suddenly. Even health-care providers, who are fully aware of the futility of reviving, strongly support out-of-hospital CPR.

The apparent contradiction between outside and inside views disappears when we see resuscitative efforts as status passage rituals, prescribed acts that provide transitions during life-changing events for those who believe in them. In analyzing status passages in another culture, the anthropologist Renato Rosaldo[38] describes the rage of bereavement that fueled the headhunting practices of the Ilongot of the Philippines:

> The raid begins with calling the spirit of the potential victim, moves through the rituals of farewell, and continues with seeking favorable omens along the trail. Most Ilongot speak about hunger and deprivation as they take days to move slowly toward the place where they will set up an ambush and await the first person who happens along. Once the raiders kill their victim, they toss away the head rather than keep it as a trophy. Before a raid, men describe their inner state by saying that the burdens of life have made them heavy and entangled, like a tree with vines clinging on it. After a successful raid, they say that they become light of step and ruddy in complexion. The collective energy of the celebration with its song, music and dance is said to give the participants a sense of well-being. This ritual process involves cleansing and catharsis.

Rosaldo analyzes this headhunting ritual as the intersection of the turmoil experienced by young Ilongot men coming of age and the raging grief experienced by elderly men who lose someone to whom they were closely attached. Faced with the accidental death of his own wife during fieldwork, Rosaldo notes in his journal his "wish for the Ilongot solution; they are much more in touch with reality than Christians. So, I need a place to carry my anger—and can we say a solution of the imagination is better than theirs?"[39] As a Christian faced with sudden death, Rosaldo longed for a way to express and make sense of his grief. Rosaldo contended that compared with the Ilongot rituals, our contemporary times seem to come up short.[40] Just as headhunting is "a solution of the imagination," a resuscitative effort is a contemporary social performance in which technological magic and suspended disbelief facilitate the transition from life to death and provide meaning to a death. It is our way of dealing with the unexpectedness of sudden death.

During some resuscitative efforts, the absurdity of reviving an obviously dead patient becomes so apparent that the emergency staff recognizes the ritualistic and performative aspects of their intervention. Once I asked a doctor at the end of a reviving attempt why he had ordered an extra chest X-ray and round of drugs (which added at least fifteen minutes to the effort). He replied:

> I wanted to buy some time. It is not as much as what happened here [in the resuscitation room] but the family. They needed time to scramble their thoughts together. This guy had a bypass and a big aneurysm. His cousin was a paramedic and started compressions right away. Then the firemen defibrillated him. In a normal case, we would have saved the patient, but not in his condition. He was already seeing a cardiologist back in [city]. I don't need to manage the patient, but I need to manage the family and give them time. This is just a ritual. A waste of time. It's a crazy world out here.

Resuscitative efforts do not necessarily save many lives, but they do provide invaluable effects for those people involved in the dying process:

• Although reviving protocols do not include opportunities for contemplating the end of life, a resuscitative effort takes some of the suddenness of sudden death away. It creates a temporal reprieve so that the bereaved can come to terms with the difficult process of dying. The actions of rescuers and paramedics provide a sense of order when death looms. For relatives and staff alike, the resuscitative effort provides an emotional distance from the devastation of sudden death.

- Despite what critics of medical technology argue, early resuscitative attempts and the administration of CPR by relatives and bystanders is definitely a community enterprise. The reviving ritual rests on the willingness of strangers to engage in intimate and potentially risky behavior. Resuscitative attempts are one of the prime secular instances that foster a sense of interpersonal solidarity. The act of putting one's mouth on the mouth of a relative or stranger and massaging that person's chest creates a close bond between rescuer and victim. Trying to save another person's life is invariably highly valued; it is associated with heroism and rewarded with medals and favorable notices in the press.
- In the hospital, the relatives and friends of a deceased person have the opportunity to talk to a social worker or chaplain who is trained in dealing with death and grieving. The institutional setting provides more personalized professional help than grievers might expect if their loved one had died suddenly at home. Professionals can also help address the logistical questions related to funerals and wills.
- Finally, and most important, the reviving effort allows relatives to conclude that everything medically possible has been done to revive their loved one. The failure of the resuscitative effort to reverse the dying process underscores the inevitability of death. The boundaries of medical power have been reached. As many relatives and staff say to console one another, "It was out of our hands." A nurse gave me a last reason why we should keep resuscitating: "It gives us the feeling that at least we have done something. We have done everything possible." Medical confirmation of death's inevitability and the opportunity for organ donation might ease survivors' guilt.[41]

With all those "side effects" of CPR, which are difficult, if not impossible, to accomplish in another way, resuscitative efforts simply do not really need to save many lives. They need only to keep the focus on lifesaving when sudden death threatens. Sally F. Moore and Barbara Myerhoff[42] commented on this aspect of secular rituals: "Ritual veils the ultimate disorder. The very thing which [the people who engage in rituals] explicitly banish is by implication their central concern." The promise that sudden death might be reversible creates sufficient order to ease the transition. And, of course, if the patient survives, the promise has been fulfilled. Whether or not a resuscitative effort saves lives, a process of identity transformation is common to all reviving attempts.

In most cases, patients make the transition from being alive to being dead. In a few, they make the transition to a chronic cardiac patient or an accident survivor.

These unexpected benefits of our instrumentalist attitude toward sudden death are particularly prominent when friends and relatives first administer CPR to the patient and when the physician makes a final decision about the condition of the patient at the end of a reviving attempt. At these two points in the resuscitation process, the needs of the relatives, friends, and even bystanders are as relevant as the urge to save lives. People who try to revive have a personal and emotional stake in the effort. Both the reviving process and its outcome matter. Through their actions, they establish a sense of control over a life-and-death situation and need to take personal responsibility for the choices they make. In those instances, the patient is not just a sum of vital indicators but a person with ties to a community. If the patient's needs and the needs of those who care are recognized, a resuscitative effort can resonate deeply in our secular culture, which has been grappling with giving meaning to sudden death. Although we still erroneously believe that all deaths can be avoided through instrumental means, resuscitative efforts can foster unity in the face of life's finality.

If we accept that resuscitative efforts "work" on a cultural level even if they do not save many lives, we need to consider whether this is the best possible way to come to terms with sudden death. What is the cost we pay with our penchant for non-lifesaving resuscitative efforts? Some of the cost is very specific to reviving. Because of the prevalence and widespread use of resuscitative efforts, it is very difficult not to be resuscitated, even if a person so chooses. To address the omnipotence of the reviving industry, we have created ambiguous legal statutes such as advance directives, living wills, DNR codes, and powers of attorney. I will show in the next chapter that these choices are often violated by the sweeping power of the resuscitative endeavor.

The more general price we pay for our over-reliance on resuscitative efforts is the increasing medicalization of death and dying. This development is particularly problematic when paramedics arrive and when the patient is transferred to the ED. Then and there, sudden death is solidly under the jurisdiction of medical professionals, excluding alternative meanings and needs. In contrast, health-care advocates have challenged views of birthing as a pathological process. For people dying a sudden death, however, the end of life remains a complex disease pat-

tern with a specific etiology that requires treatment and medical attendance. The person is not just dying at the end of the life course; he or
she can become "a pulmonary embolism [that] caused a fatal cerebral
vascular accident." This far-reaching medicalization of death is evident
in the national bestseller *How We Die*, by Sherwin Nuland,[43] who details
the biological and clinical processes that underlie the most common
ways of dying while disregarding the social and emotional impact of
dying. As Nancy Scheper-Hughes and Margaret M. Lock explain, "medicalization inevitably entails a missed identification between the individual and the social bodies, and a tendency to transform the social into
the biological."[44] Charis Cussins noted in her analysis of infertility treatments that medicalization is not experienced as problematic when the
expected result is obtained, but it becomes a source of violation, objec-
tification, bureaucratization, and loss of self and agency when the
promised result is lacking.[45]

Medicalization of dying and the consequent exclusion of relatives
and friends from the central part of the resuscitation process are particularly unfortunate. While the patient is resuscitated in the ED, relatives and bystanders—who may well have instigated the resuscitative effort through CPR and who saw paramedics trying to revive the
patient—are whisked off to a counseling or family room. They generally do not know what has happened to their loved one until a physician, nurse, or chaplain informs them that the patient is now dead.
Even when they are allowed to greet the deceased body, the signs of
the dying process and the reviving effort have been removed, and the
body appears to be sleeping. Death as a final state is visible, but the
process of dying occurred in secret, backstage, removed from the audience that ultimately cares the most. The defining moment of the entire resuscitation ritual is not significant for the staff, who have only
professional ties to the patient, but it might mean everything to relatives and friends.[46]

Above all, resuscitative efforts in the ED perpetuate the dominant position of the medical professionals. Theirs is the final decision authority over when and whether a person is dead. Like all monopolies over
body practices, this power poses a potential danger because medical
professionals become the sole agents of social control. They are in the
position to define what is a good death and a bad death, good grieving
and bad grieving, and most important, which lives are worth saving and
which are not. In the next chapter, I will explore the consequences of re-

lying on medical professionals to facilitate the transition between life and death. There I take a closer look at the decision-making process during reviving efforts.

5   Deciding Life and Death

REACHING DECISIONS

IN 1967, the sociologist David Sudnow offered the following advice: "If you anticipate having a critical heart attack, keep yourself well-dressed and your breath clean."[1] Sudnow was the first to note that whether a patient lives or dies at the end of a resuscitative effort depends to a certain extent on the emergency department staff's interpretation of striking social characteristics—such as the patient's age, "moral character," and clinical teaching value. The staff regarded certain groups of people as "socially dead," meaning that "a patient is treated essentially as a corpse, though perhaps still 'clinically' and 'biologically' alive."[2] Sudnow explained that

> two persons in "similar" physical condition may be differentially designated dead or not. For example, a young child was brought into the ER with no registering heartbeat, respirations, or pulse—the standard "signs of death"—and was, through a rather dramatic stimulation procedure involving the coordinated work of a large team of doctors and nurses, revived for a period of eleven hours. On the same evening, shortly after the child's arrival, an elderly person who presented the same physical signs, with what a doctor later stated, in conversation, to be no discernible differences from the child in skin color, warmth, etc., "arrived" in the ER and was almost immediately pronounced dead, with no attempts at stimulation instituted.

The most disturbing aspect of Sudnow's analysis was his conclusion that social death became a predictor for biological death during resuscitative attempts. The ED staff was less likely to attempt resuscitating "the suicide victim, the dope addict, the known prostitute, the assailant in a crime of violence, the vagrant, the known wife-beater, and, generally, those persons whose moral character are considered reproachable."[3]

Zygmunt Bauman[4] recently questioned whether Sudnow's observations are still relevant.[5] He postulated that because resuscitative efforts have "lost much of their specularity and have ceased to impress, their discriminating power has all but dissipated."[6] The members of a hospital's institutional review board echoed this sentiment when I originally asked permission to observe the decision-making process during resuscitative efforts. They assured me that decision making is an "irrelevant" question because "they just followed the protocols."[7] Indeed, since Sudnow studied hospital dying in the early sixties, two important developments have changed the health-care landscape. First, the rationalization of medical knowledge has promised to turn the "art" of medical practice into a "science"[8] and eliminate the social problems of experimental medical technology. Biomedical researchers have interpreted clinical decision making in terms of formal probabilistic reasoning and algorithms that link clinical data inputs with therapeutic decision outputs.[9] According to this view, health-care providers reach decisions during lifesaving efforts simply by following the resuscitation protocols until they run into an end point. The data they consider consists solely of observable clinical parameters and biomedical test results.

Second, legislators have made it obligatory for health-care providers to initiate CPR whenever medically indicated.[10] Once the emergency medical system is alerted, health-care providers have the legal and ethical duty to continue resuscitating until the protocols are exhausted. At the same time, ethicists and legislators have tried to increase and protect patient autonomy. The Patient Self-Determination Act of 1991[11] mandated that patients be given notice of their rights to make medical-treatment decisions and of the legal instruments available to give force to decisions made in advance. This attempt at de-medicalizing[12] sudden death again is indirectly aimed at diminishing social rationing, the deliberate withholding of potentially beneficial medical care. When patients have decided that they do not want to be resuscitated, the staff should follow the written directives regardless of the patient's social value.

The sociological literature of the sixties suggests that in the past, health-care providers alternated between resuscitating aggressively and preparing for impending death on the basis of the patient's social viability. In contrast, legislators and biomedical researchers have now designed an emergency system in which care providers are required to save lives whenever medically indicated. Now, only people who choose not to be resuscitated should be exempt from a reviving attempt. ED staff should no longer systematically withhold potentially beneficial care from groups with a low social value. To do so would mean passive euthanasia for some and aggressive but futile lifesaving efforts with needless suffering for others, whose presumed social value is higher. The question, then, is whether resuscitation protocols and legal protections, instituted since the sixties, have in fact eliminated the social inequality that Sudnow observed.

INITIAL IMPRESSION

Decision making depends on available information, but every patient who enters the ED in cardiac arrest is initially unknown to the staff. Still, the resuscitation team does not start a reviving effort with a blank slate. The staff receives the first clues about the patient's condition when the paramedics radio the ED of their impending arrival.[13] These reports follow a standard format. The paramedics first describe the main complaint, which, in cases of resuscitation, is full cardiac arrest. At that time, the person taking the call, usually a nurse, informs the departmental administrator that a "level-one medical" or a "code blue" is on the way. While the administrator pages the medical staff, the paramedics continue their report with the standard phrase, "On arrival at the scene, we found the patient ..." followed by details of the circumstances of the cardiopulmonary arrest. For example, in one observation, the paramedics reported, "On arrival at the scene, we found the patient lying down in front of her class. Patient fell down ten minutes before arrival, and CPR was started right away." The paramedics then describe the patient's biomedical condition. They mention the vital signs—blood pressure, electrocardiac rhythm, pulse, breathing rate and quality—and the level of consciousness. If there was time for treatment, or if changes have occurred in the vital parameters, the paramedics update these indicators and report reactions during the radio call. Sometimes they provide demographic information such as the patient's sex, race, and age. The radio call ends with the ETA, or estimated time of arrival.

On the basis of the few clues they have from the circumstances of the cardiopulmonary arrest, the social characteristics, the biomedical indicators, and the treatment, the medical staff forms an initial impression. Team members have two important questions. First, does the patient have a reasonable chance of survival? Second, how long will we work on the patient? The health-care staff estimates the probability of survival. In some cases, the staff leaves the margin of viability open, perhaps because adequate information is unavailable to assess or because some indicators contradict one another. But in many situations, combinations of circumstantial and biomedical information provide a definitive assessment. An example from my observations:

The paramedic reported over the radio, "Patient was found in cornfields. Nobody knows how long he has been down. Patient was last seen three hours before being found. Patient has no pulse, no respirations, totally unresponsive, asystole." Ruth Berns, the nurse taking this message, turned around to the secretary and told her, "You can call the coroner."

The notice of an unwitnessed arrest contained enough information for Berns to conclude that the patient was biologically dead and that any resuscitation attempt would be futile.

After the radio report, the staff usually has a few minutes to prepare for the arrival of the ambulance. With the previously mentioned information in mind, the staff anticipate the time they will spend on the patient. The resuscitation might be a routine fifteen-minute ritual, or it might occupy two nurses and a physician for several hours. For example,

> I am paged while reading. When I enter the ED, the secretary directs me to room seven. The patient hasn't arrived yet. I ask Miriam Fallows (a nurse), "What's the story?" She answers, "A 75-year-old lady. Diabetic, asthmatic. They gave two epis and two atropines. She went from JVD to V-fib, and is now in asystole." She adds, "It will be a short one." A little later, a nurse from intensive care enters, but Miriam sends her back, saying, "We will not need you."

In this case, the nurse in charge of the shift assigned the patient to a primary nurse and a back-up nurse. One of the nurses informed an emergency physician of the patient's impending arrival and delegated tasks to the remaining staff. Their initial impression was that the resuscitative effort would not take very long and would end with a deceased patient.

The staff keeps this initial impression in mind for the patient's arrival. An initial impression is rather fragile, however, and many elements might require adjustment. The patient might be the same, worse, or better than the medical staff originally thought. The nurse answering the call might not have written down all the relevant information; the paramedics might not have had time to give a full report; their measurements might have been inaccurate because of the moving ambulance or they might not have known the exact biomedical information. In other cases, the patient might have been brought by car or might have had a cardiopulmonary arrest while already in the ED.

DEAD ON ARRIVAL

Occasionally, the physician reaches a final decision the moment the patient arrives in the ED, so that the patient is declared "DOA," or "dead on arrival." I observed DOA only when an extraordinarily long transportation time had occurred and all the possible drugs had been given to a patient who remained unresponsive. For example,

> Dr. Richard Hendrickson takes me aside before the patient arrives and says, "Stefan, I just want to tell you that the patient has been down for more than half an hour [before the paramedics arrived]. They had a long ride. I probably will declare the patient dead on arrival." When the patient arrives, the paramedic reports, "We had asystole for the last ten minutes. We think he was in V-fib for a while, but it was en route. It could have been the movement of the ambulance." The physician replies, "I declare this patient dead."

In the early sixties, David Sudnow noted that DOA was the most common dying scenario in EDs. Legal changes have now diminished the importance of the DOA trajectory. When someone calls 911, a resuscitative effort begins and is virtually unstoppable until a physician sees the patient in the ED. After the rescue call, an ambulance with EMTs or paramedics is dispatched. Unless the patient shows obvious signs of death,[14] the ambulance rescuers need to start the CPR and ACLS treatment as prescribed by their standing orders and protocols. Implied consent is assumed for this treatment.[15] The patient is thus transported to the ED, where the physician with the resuscitation team takes over. Legally, the physician again cannot stop the lifesaving attempt because he or she needs to make sure that the protocols are exhausted. Stopping sooner would qualify as negligence and be grounds for malpractice.

THE RUSH OF THE FIRST MINUTES

The Resuscitation Team

In most cases, the ED team is legally obligated to continue the resuscitation attempt started by the paramedics. A few seconds after the patient is rolled into the emergency room, four to eight health-care providers work simultaneously. To create some order in the crawling of bodies, spatial positions correlate with the tasks of each team member.

The patient lies face up in the center of the room. The patient's head is directed toward the back wall. Above the head and attached to the ceiling hangs a heart monitor. The respiratory therapist stands between the patient's head and the wall, hands rhythmically squeezing the ventilation bag. The technician is positioned on a little stool to the left of the patient. The technician's hips lean above the patient's chest. In that position, the technicians can give chest compressions using their body weight.

The physician initially stands close to the patient's head, between the respiratory therapist and the emergency technician. From that spot, the physician is able to perform a variety of tasks. If the patient has not been intubated, the physician can intubate, feel for a radial pulse, check the pupils, oscillate for breath sounds, and, if necessary, establish a central line in the patient's neck.

One nurse, usually the nurse in charge, stands at one of the patient's arms to connect an IV lifeline, administer intravenous medication, or defibrillate the patient. The nurse also attaches the patches of the ED heart monitor to the patient's chest. A second respiratory therapist or a phlebologist takes blood from an artery in the groin. The back-up nurse oversees the action and takes notes at the feet of the patient. Two other people—nurses, paramedics, or technicians—walk around. They remove drugs from boxes and hand these to the nurse or administer the drugs themselves. They are also messengers, walking back and forth between the emergency room and administrator, relatives, or chaplain and supplying the emergency room with missing items.

Retrieving Clinical Information

During the first minutes, when the patient is carefully moved from the ambulance stretcher to the ED bed, every professional connects the patient to artificial lifesaving devices and monitors. With the patient's presence, the process of determining how much resuscitative care is sufficient escalates. The patient's general appearance contains hundreds of possible clues, but the medical staff makes only the relevant clues visible. Mike Lynch calls this aspect of patient care "turning up signs": "The patient was not a Rosetta stone, a surface upon which signs could already be seen to be inscribed."[16] Turning up signs means that retrieving information also involves attending to some data and obfuscating other indicators. Clues become informative when the staff considers them representative of the patient's condition. For example, one patient I observed had a huge bulk of scar tissue from a gunshot wound sticking about a foot out of the stomach area. The staff ignored this very visible deformity throughout the resuscitative effort.

The patient's color, temperature, and smell are important indicators of the his or her condition. Dark purple ears, mottled extremities, or dusky gray fingernails are signs of inadequate tissue perfusion and possible biological death. Color is closely related to the patient's temperature. One does not need a thermometer; the mere touch of the body tells the health-care provider whether the body is very cold or still rather warm. Depending on the weather outside, a cold or warm body increases or decreases the patient's viability. Nurse Marie Rivers explained, "If it is a hypothermic patient, the body slows down. They have a cooling factor involved. You can try to rewarm the patient. Of course, the patients that lock themselves in their trailer and leave the gas on and put the furnace on as hard as they can and then overdose and go into cardiac arrest, those are usually the ones that don't come back because they have the extra heat on." Warming produces a faint but definite smell of biological decay in progress. Sometimes a patient's medical condition is apparent from the general appearance, as for a patient with a dialysis catheter sticking out of the belly. In other cases, the overview provides clues about the circumstances of the cardiac arrest: a patient in a swimsuit, evening gown, pajamas, or golf shoes.

The attention of the medical practitioners usually shifts from appearances to the more specialized indicators of the patient's condition. The respiratory therapists focus on breathing. The resistance that the respiratory therapist encounters while squeezing the oxygen reservoir provides information about the condition of the lungs. If the lungs are congested, the respiratory therapist needs to push harder, and the result is less productive. The respiratory therapist who takes a blood sample from an artery also receives an indirect but strong indicator of the patient's condition. Without enough blood pressure to fill a tube with blood, or with blood that is dark blue to black in color, the team can identify insufficient blood circulation or oxygenation.

One of the main signifiers of the patient's condition is the electrocardiac heart (EKG) rhythm. The electric current flowing through the heart is constantly visible as a characteristic orange or green line on a display screen. Regularly, medical staff check this screen and make decisions based on the pattern of the line. The emergency technician notes the effect of the chest compressions by observing the impact on the

heart rhythm. Nurses and the physician also check the monitor for unusual heart rhythms.

In medical handbooks and protocols, the EKG rhythm is portrayed
as such a crucial indicator of the patient's clinical viability that the books
include the admonition to "treat the patient, not the monitor."[17] Basically, when the monitor shows a persistent flat line (asystole) or a prolonged pulseless anginal rhythm in different leads, the patient is biologically dead. When the line on the monitor displays certain regular
patterns, the patient is stabilized. My observations of resuscitative attempts indicate, however, that cardiac rhythms are neither a sufficient
nor a necessary condition for an aggressive reviving attempt or an official pronouncement of death. The health-care providers I observed
did not always trust the rhythm, especially when they suspected an
anomalous result. Compressions of the technician, respiratory manipulation, bumping into the bed of the patient, a loose electrode, an internal pacemaker, or an empty battery in the portable monitor can all
influence the electrical rhythm.

But even after ambiguity is ruled out, the staff does not aggressively
revive all clinically viable patients. Neither does the staff give up on all
biologically dead patients. For example, in many of the resuscitative efforts I witnessed, a flat line was present when the patient arrived in the
ED, but the medical staff still attempted to resuscitate for ten to twenty
minutes while the cardiac rhythm remained unchanged. In other observations, the monitor showed a regular and recognizable heart
rhythm. Still, the medical staff did not consider the patient stabilized and
instead expected the rhythm to change to asystole. In one resuscitative
attempt, the patient was connected to two monitors that showed different rhythms. As I observed,

> The patient arrived in the ED attached to a portable monitor
> with the possibility of automatic defibrillation (electric shock-
> ing). The ED staff attached the patient to their own monitor but
> kept the patient on the portable monitor. This meant that the pa-
> tient was attached to two different monitors, which showed two
> slightly different rhythms. In the early moments of the resuscita-
> tion, the medical staff focused on the more "optimistic" heart
> rhythm of the portable monitor, but when it became clear that
> the resuscitative endeavor was futile, the attention shifted to the
> ED monitor, and the portable monitor was switched off.

In this case, the physician and nurse resolved the issue of different rhythms by switching monitors when their definition of the situation changed. The EKG rhythm, as pre-interpreted in protocols and guidelines, was not self-evident; it needed to be managed and contextualized with details about the pre-hospital resuscitative effort and the patient's presumed social viability. While clinical information is retrieved and exchanged, the paramedics debrief the nurse responsible for taking notes. That person sifts through all the details and documents the indicators relevant for the patient's assessment and necessary for record keeping. The notetaker asks the paramedics specific questions about the circumstances of the arrest. When exactly was the patient down? When did they receive the radio call? Who started CPR?

Circumstances of the Cardiac Arrest

The staff interprets the information about the circumstances of the cardiac arrest in light of the dominant resuscitation theory. Physicians, nurses, technicians, and ED chaplains reiterated the basics of resuscitation theory: the more quickly the steps in the "chain of survival" are carried out,[18] the better the chances for survival (see Figure 3-3). A weakness in one step will reverberate throughout the entire system and impair optimal survival rates. The chain consists of four links: early notification of the emergency system, early CPR, early defibrillation, and early drug therapy. Ideally, the time span between the patient's collapse and the fourth step should not exceed five minutes, because otherwise irreversible brain damage might develop.

The professional rescuers in the ED are acutely aware of their location in the chain of survival. The ED is the last link, and much needs to be in place before the patient reaches the team. Anything that deviates from the "ideal" resuscitative pattern and causes more time to elapse is a matter of concern. Josh Brittan, a technician, estimated the importance of every step for the outcome:

> One of the most important things would be the time between when the patient actually went down until the first people arrive. That is like, I'd say, 30 percent, and then the time that a patient takes to get to the hospital probably takes another 30 to 40 percent; 60 to 70 percent of it is pre-hospital time.

Nurse Judith Kaufert explained the importance of location and timing by contrasting resuscitating inside and outside the ED:

A lot has to do with EMS [emergency medical system] and family response and getting them here. If you would drop dead right here, your chances would be pretty good that we would be able to resuscitate you without any brain damage or anything else. If you're at home out on a farm, sixty miles away, and you have to call out for help, and that takes fifteen minutes for them to get there, and nobody in the house knows CPR, I think your chances are pretty slim.

According to Kaufert, if first steps have not been optimal, the ED staff cannot be expected to rectify the situation. Health-care providers are less willing to resuscitate patients aggressively when they have deviated from the ideal scenario. The technician Adam Dinkes noted that, in many cases, he "start[s] to feel already defeated—to the point now where resuscitations I see coming into the ER it is pretty much decided already, we are not going to get anywhere with this." Thus, even if the patient has reasonably good clinical indicators, the staff may believe that dying has progressed to the point that intervention is useless. Therefore, when paramedics tell the staff that a cardiac arrest was unwitnessed, that they had a long transportation time, that CPR was done by a nonprofessional, that they could not defibrillate the patient, that they could not establish intravenous lines, or that the patient was already asystolic at their arrival, the chances of survival are not only diminished but the staff also might not want to revive the patient. Their fear is brain damage.

The Patient's Social Viability

Clinical observations also reflect the patient's social characteristics. Certain outstanding social characteristics have significant moral connotations that affect the intensity with which the staff approaches the resuscitative effort. The most outstanding social characteristics are age and the perceived seriousness of the illness. These variables, of course, also have medical meanings, but the strong value judgments about the patient's quality of life—present and future—attached to age and perceived seriousness of the illness render these variables social. Their normativeness is not medically defensible.

In essence, ED staff are more willing to revive young, healthy patients than elderly or seriously ill patients. For example, Nurse Mark Lanchester explained to me that older people would want to die: "Maybe this 80-year-old guy just fell over at home, and maybe that is the way he wanted to go. But no, somebody calls an ambulance and brings him to the ER, where we work and work and work and get him to the in-tensive-care unit, where he is poked and prodded for a few days, and then they finally decide to let him go." According to Nurse Jennifer Cohen, older people have nothing more to live for: "People [who] are in their seventies, eighties, have lived their lives, but people, young people who experience sudden death, those [resuscitative efforts] are difficult." In contrast, young children should not die. Nurse Ruth Berns explained that a child's death "goes against the scheme of things. Par-ents are not supposed to bury their children. The children are supposed to bury their parents." Physician David Reznikov noted: "You are nat-urally more aggressive with younger people. If I had a 40-year-old who had a massive MI [myocardial infarction], was asystolic for twenty min-utes, or something like that, I would be very aggressive with that per-son. I suppose for the same scenario with a 90-year-old, I might not be." A colleague agreed: "When you have a younger patient, you try to give it a little bit more effort. You might want to go another half-hour on a younger person because you have such a difficult time letting the per-son go." Although respondents hesitated to give me an age cut-off point, all agreed that the resuscitation of young people triggered an aggres-sive lifesaving attempt.

Serious illness, in turn, is equated with suffering. When a patient has lived with a serious illness, sudden death might be considered a bless-ing. The hospital chaplain Rick Heller gave me an example: "In some instances, we may not be worse off, but we may not be better off [with CPR]. This occurs when a person is suffering from a terminal condition, and death is relatively imminent anyway." The staff pities terminally ill patients and hopes that their passing is painless. Health-care providers find out about the medical history from paramedics, relatives, and pa-tients charts, or from scars and other body marks.

In addition to age and health status, the staff takes into account an-other group of valuable patients—those the staff recognizes because of their prominence in the community. In some cases, the entire resuscita-tive team might know the patient; in other cases, the patient reminds one or several team members of someone they know. The resuscitative effort of a well-known sports coach or a prominent politician is different be-cause of the patient's highly visible position in the community at large. For example, I learned of a well-liked and well-known senior hospital employee who was resuscitated. All the respondents involved made extensive reference to this particular resuscitative effort. When I asked Dave Johnson, a respiratory therapist, how this effort differed from the others, he replied, "I think the routines and procedures were the same, but I think the sense of urgency was a lot greater. The anxiety level was higher. We were more tense. It was very different from, say, a 98-year-old from a nursing home."

Staff also respond aggressively to patients with whom they identify. Nurse Cohen reflected, "Incidentally, any time there is an association of a resuscitation with something that you have a close relationship with—your family, the age range, the situation . . . there is more emotional involvement." The identifiable patient receives a kind of personhood because of a very striking characteristic, such as belonging to the same age group or resembling the physical countenance of one's children, a partner, parents, or close friends of the care provider. Cohen told me how she broke down after performing a thoracotomy and open-heart cardiac massage on a teenage patient while her own children were teenagers. Recognition can also be more subtle. Another nurse explained how a resuscitative effort became more difficult after she had established a relationship with the patient by talking to her and carrying out the routine patient-assessment procedures.

Age and medical history have become "master traits"[19] during the resuscitative effort. The impact of other identity signifiers—such as sex, race, religion, sexual orientation, and socioeconomic status—was more difficult to note. The longest resuscitative effort I observed was performed on a person with presumably low social worth based on his socioeconomic status, a white homeless man who fell into a creek and was hypothermic. I also noticed that the staff made many disturbingly insensitive jokes during the resuscitative effort of a person with a high socioeconomic status, an apparently well-dressed and wealthy elderly white woman who had collapsed during dinner in one of the fanciest restaurants in the city. During a particularly hectic day, the staff worked very hard and long to save a middle-aged African American woman who collapsed in front of her classroom, while two white elderly men who were also brought in in cardiac arrest that day were quickly pronounced dead. Because of the low overall survival rate in my study, it is difficult to reach conclusions about the role of race, sex, religion, marital affiliation, sexual orientation, and socioeconomic status in resuscitative efforts.

Epidemiological studies, however, suggest that race, sex, and socioeconomic status play a significant role in overall survival of a sudden cardiac arrest. The emergency medical system is much more likely to be alerted when men die at home than when women experience cardiac arrest, which suggests a selection bias in the system.[20] Women also have significantly lower survival rates than men. In a Minneapolis study, the survival rate to one year after cardiac arrest was 3.5 percent for women and 13.1 percent for men.[21] A similar relationship has been observed for racial differences. Not only was the incidence of cardiac arrest in Chicago during 1988 significantly higher among blacks in every age group than among whites, but the survival rate of blacks after an out-of-hospital cardiac arrest was only a third of that among whites (1% versus 3%). But race failed to predict resuscitation outcome when controlled for income in a different study.[22] Daniel Brookoff and collaborators[23] showed that black victims of cardiac arrest receive CPR less frequently than white victims. Using tax-assessment data, Alfred Hallstrom's research team[24] demonstrated that people in lower socioeconomic strata are at a greater risk for higher mortality. In addition, lower-class people were also less likely to survive an episode of out-of-hospital cardiac arrest: "an increase of $50,000 in the valuation per unit of the home address increased the patient's chance of survival by 60%."[25] It is important to keep in mind that these studies reflect the working of the entire emergency medical system, not just that of the ED staff. Lower survival rates for racial minorities, for example, could be explained partly as a consequence of the staff's attitude toward minorities, or it could also indicate the location of hospitals in cities (farther from minority neighborhoods); different cardiac-disease incidence because of nutrition and socioeconomic status; a more suspicious attitude toward uniformed emergency personnel; and so forth. As in any study of survival rates, the operationalization of these variables should be critically analyzed.

Whenever a patient can transcend anonymity and become more than a mere body, the staff considers the person valuable, with some potential for resuscitative success. The only exception to this rule are drunks and drug addicts. They often are identifiable in the ED, but are associated with low social viability. Death is considered an "appropriate" retaliation for their condition. I observed one resuscitative attempt on a patient who had overdosed on heroin. The team went through the resuscitation motions, but without much vigor or sympathy. Instead, staff members wore double pairs of gloves, avoided touching the patient, joked about their difficulty inserting an intravenous line, and mentioned how they loathed bringing the bad news to the patient's belligerent "girlfriend."

Although I could easily observe cases in which the patient had a high perceived social viability, characteristics of low perceived social-viability were subtle. For example:

> Nurse Mabel Hall, administering the drug, says, "Well, he seems to be doing better." Ginny Kincaid, the respiratory therapist working at the head of the patient answers, "I don't think so. Look at the ears. They're getting totally purple, and see, the cornea is dried up." Marie Rivers replies, "Yes, but he feels warmer, and the IVs are running." Ken Glasser, the nurse supervisor, interferes, "I don't think he will make it. He has been down for at least half an hour and he has an extensive heart-disease history." Ginny Kincaid adds, "He is also in his seventies."

In this conversation, the patient's age was the final justification for likely death. I saw health-care professionals subscribe to a moral hierarchy in which some lives are worth living and in which for others death is the better outcome. In this way, social characteristics, in combination with other variables, affect the course of a reviving attempt.

RESUSCITATION TRAJECTORIES

When the first rush of the resuscitative effort has abated, the staff relates information about the patient's social viability, the circumstances of the cardiac arrest, and the patient's clinical viability. As the technician Josh Brittan remarked, "Later, you get the background of the patient from the nurse who was in there with the paramedics. Once you get that, you know whether you're beating a dead horse or whether you might be effective." Similar to the initial impression formed before the patient's arrival in the ED is an operational definition of the situation. Such an assessment rests again on two concerns: what is the patient's condition and prognosis, and what work is involved? Answers are evident in the drugs that the physician orders, the actions considered appropriate, and the time that staff anticipate spending with the patient. For example,

Expressing his frustration with the poor condition of the patient, Dr. Brian Waxman says, "Let's keep up this nonsense for ten minutes, and then I will call the patient [declare the patient dead]. Give one more epi[nephrine]." He leaves the room.

After the staff formulates an operational definition of the situation, four different resuscitation trajectories emerge:

1. Most patients are people with a presumed low social viability. Significant time has elapsed since they arrived in the ED, and they do not have viable clinical signs. In this scenario, death is mostly a legal matter, so I call this the *legal death trajectory*.
2. The second group consists of patients with a presumed high social viability who die at the end of the reviving effort. Whether they had a long or short transportation time or even whether they show clinical viability scarcely matters. The staff aggressively tries to save their lives. Because the patient's presumed high social status overwhelms the resuscitative effort, this is the *elite death trajectory*.
3. The third group consists of patients with assumed low social viability and a relatively short pre-hospital resuscitative effort. On arrival in the ED, however, these patients still have some clinical viability. The shape of this trajectory often resembles a roller-coaster, so I will refer to it as *temporary stabilization trajectory*.
4. The final trajectory is followed by patients with either a presumed high or a presumed low social viability. These have an exceptionally short transportation time and good clinical parameters. This situation best promotes survival, so I use the term *stabilization trajectory*.

I estimate that in my study only 3 percent of resuscitative efforts followed the last pattern. This low figure might be a slight underestimate because the stabilization trajectory occurs very quickly and is therefore difficult to observe. It is possible that the resuscitative effort was over before I was paged. The temporary stabilization trajectory occurred in about 7 percent of the lifesaving attempts. DOA occurred in about 5 percent of the resuscitative efforts. The elite death trajectory explained an estimated 10 percent of the cases I observed. Finally, the legal death trajectory was the most common, occurring in about 75 percent of the observed resuscitation attempts. Of the 112 resuscitative efforts that I observed, only eleven patients were stabilized at the end. Of those, I know of only one patient who survived for several months. Some of the other ten died after a couple of days or remained in a comatose condition until life support was switched off. Because I could not always follow these patients, I am not sure how many survived for a significant period. I do know that the staff in the ED did not expect most of the stabilized patients to walk out of the hospital.

In the ED, sudden death is thus a combination of clinical, biological, social, and legal factors. Clinical death occurs when the signs of death first become apparent: when breathing ceases and the pulse disappears. At that point, a small window of opportunity remains in which the organic dying process can be reversed. Biological death is the end point of the clinical dying process. It is irreversible. A patient is socially dead when others (the staff, relatives, and friends) consider the person to be deceased and act toward the person as a deceased human being. Legal death refers to the official pronounciation of death; it occurs when the physician officially terminates the reviving attempt and notes the time of death. At the beginning of resuscitative efforts in the ED, every patient is presumed to be clinically dead. The sequence of biological, social, and legal death distinguish the different resuscitation trajectories.

Legal Death Trajectory

During the vast majority of resuscitative efforts, the staff considers the patient already deceased while they perform the "lifesaving" procedures. In a typical situation, the physician tells the team at 7:55 A.M. that the patient will be dead at 8:05 A.M. The physician then leaves to fill out paperwork or talk to the patient's relatives. Exactly at 8:05, the team stops the effort; the nurse responsible for taking notes writes down the time of death; and the team disperses. In two resuscitative efforts, I observed that the staff even called the coroner while resuscitating.

The prevalence of these cases is largely a consequence of the structure of the emergency system and legal requirements. Paramedics need to follow standing orders to resuscitate and transport the patient to the ED, where a physician is present. The physician has the authority to declare the patient dead, but only after the resuscitation protocols have been exhausted. Stopping sooner would qualify as abandonment and might expose the physician and hospital to malpractice charges. The kind of insurance the patient carries further determines the length of a resuscitative effort (some insurers require minimum resuscitation lengths). In most cases, therefore, the physician orders at least one more round of drugs, checks whether the patient is correctly intubated, glances at the EKG rhythm, maybe implants a central intravenous line in the jugular vein, and waits for any reactions.

Two categories of patients follow this trajectory: patients who are obviously biologically dead and those who might still be biologically viable but are deemed socially dead. Referring to the lack of cardiac and respiratory functioning, staff often call patients who seem biologically dead "pulseless non-breathers," "goners," or "flatliners." Most of those patients are elderly or suffer from serious illnesses. Babies who have died from sudden infant death syndrome and some young adults might also be pulseless non-breathers, but because they are deemed valuable and viable, the staff does not include them in this group. The respiratory therapist Ginny Kincaid described her reaction to the flatliners: "If it comes over my beeper that there is a pulseless non-breather, then I know they were at home. I know that they were down a long time.... I go and do my thing. It's over when they get here." Some respondents added that this group did not leave a lasting impression: "They all blend together as one gray blur." Although medical researchers confirm that patients who arrive in the ED without a pulse have almost no chance of functional recovery,[26] legal requirements stipulate that pulseless non-breathers need resuscitative motions. Such a prolonged resuscitative attempt does not necessarily mean that the staff believes these people have a chance to revive or even that the staff wants to revive them.

In several such resuscitative efforts, the nurses and technicians envied the quickness of sudden death. When I entered the resuscitation room on a rainy May evening, Nurse Jennifer Cohen took me aside and told me, "I don't know if this is useful for your research, but I buried my dad two days ago." I replied, "Oh, I'm sorry. Is this difficult for you?" "No, at least [the patient] didn't have to be in a vegetative state for two months like my dad." Technician Maggie Linquist, who overheard us, added, "Or eighteen months, like my dad." In several resuscitative efforts, the nurses looked at the patient they were "resuscitating" and confided to one another: "This is how I would like to die. Boom, death. In one time,"[27] or "At least it was quick and sweet."

But not all patients who follow this trajectory are biologically dead. Some are still biologically viable but considered socially dead. Even when the staff expects these patients to die, the signs of life might still return. The elderly or seriously ill patient might unexpectedly regain a pulse or start breathing. This development is often an unsettling discovery and poses a dilemma: are we going to try to "save" this patient, or will we let the patient die? In all my observations of patients already deemed socially dead, such signs of life were disregarded or explained away, especially when people not in charge of the resuscitative effort observed a pulse or renewed breathing. A physician in charge who notices signs of life can consider them important and continue the resuscitative effort. The physician has more power than the other members of the resuscitation team to institute and validate reality.[28] Therefore, the first way to explain away signs of life is to refer implicitly to the inexperience of the person making the observation:

> The EMT-A who has a stethoscope listens for heart sounds and says, "I heard a bump. I don't know if it was the machine or the patient." Then Nurse Judith Kaufert listens. She says she also hears weak heart tones. But she doubts if she really hears them. "It can be my imagination or wishful thinking." Finally, Physician John Cole listens and then shakes his head. "No heart tones. Wait for a flat line and then hook off the ventilator." He leaves the room.

Nurses and technicians are not the only ones who "imagine" life where death seems to be established. In the case of the heroin overdose, the monitor suddenly indicated a palpable blood pressure while the patient was in asystole. The doctor disregarded the blood pressure, saying, "The machine has an imagination of its own."

Another way to dismiss signs of life is to redefine them as artifacts of the resuscitation process. The artificial means of maintaining life could confuse staff about the viability of the patient. To qualify as real indicators of life, the signs need to be sustained apart from the lifesaving actions. The staff therefore checks the EKG monitor after pausing with chest compressions because the mere pressing of the chest distorts the EKG rhythm. At the same time, however, respiratory therapists would continue artificial ventilation with a mask and bag device, which offers a convenient alternative explanation for any signs of life. At the end of one resuscitative effort, a nurse drew the team's attention to the monitor, where an irregular wavy line was visible. A colleague replied, "I am afraid that's [respiratory therapist] Jennifer's bagging."

The staff also relies on biomedical theory to explain away the sudden development of life signs, usually after the physician has declared the patient dead or has determined to do so:

At 18:57 the patient is declared dead, and the two respiratory therapists leave. We put the sheet over the patient, but Josh Brittan (the technician) and I stop suddenly: the sheet goes up and down over the patient's torso. We bring this to the attention of Suzy Danvers (a nurse). She takes off the sheet and listens for heart sounds. "I hear some, but I can't palpate them."

Brittan runs to get Dr. Brian Waxman. Danvers keeps listening and looks at the monitor. The physician enters. Danvers says, "I hear heart tones. Is this the medication?" Waxman looks at the almost straight line and says half jokingly, "You should not have listened." Danvers answers, "Don't say that doctor. Now I'll have nightmares about Dr. Waxman telling me not to listen." They both laugh, then the physician asks, "Has it been fifteen minutes? Then I declare the patient deceased." He looks at the rising of the chest and says: "This should stop before the coroner gets here." Again everyone laughs, "People don't die like in the movies, right?" "Right," answers Brittan. Dr. Waxman continues, "If you die, it's your heart, your lungs, or both. This is just his toxic reflex. His brainstem is still working. It will probably stop pretty soon."

In a similar situation, a nurse dismissed the patient's breathing without a heartbeat by declaring, "That is an animal instinct, a reflex."

The same reasoning applies when the staff suspects that the patient has suffered from extensive brain damage. In those situations, the staff tries explicitly not to revive the patient. One nurse admonished her colleagues during a resuscitative effort for Richard Elmer, the patient who had collapsed during an award ceremony: "Take it easy," she advised, "Don't do anything. He will for sure be brain dead by now. We don't want to do that to the man of the year." In another situation, Dr. Brian Waxman was even more blunt:

The physician re-enters the resuscitation room. He asks, "Got rid of that pulse yet?" He sees me and explains, "She had all kinds of cancer. They were stupid enough not to ask for a red alert, and now we have to go through this nonsense."

Staff members refer to resuscitating as "running a code." When social death has preceded biological death or biological death has preceded legal death, the staff still "runs" the code but really "walks" it slowly.[29]

In other words, the team goes through the motions but tries explicitly not to get a pulse back. Resuscitation staff refer to those lukewarm CPR attempts as "partial, slow, light, blue, or Hollywood" codes.[30]

Because they consider the reviving efforts futile, health-care providers use the time for other purposes. While they are compressing the chest and artificially ventilating the patient, conversation drifts to other topics such as birthday parties, television shows, hunting events, sports, awful patients, staffing conflicts, and easy or difficult shifts. During one resuscitative effort, nurses exchanged ideas for birthday parties for 6-year-old-girls, while in a different reviving attempt a technician and paramedics discussed a recent Dolly Parton show and the price of used hunting guns.

During legal death resuscitative trajectories, staff members often joke about the patient, about themselves, or about the absurdness of the situation. Looking at a deceased patient's pale feet, a technician remarked, "Well, I think he can use some more sun." When a physician who stood too close to the patient during a defibrillation attempt was kicked in the groin by the twisting body, he chirped, "From now on, I'll talk with a high voice." When a nurse administrator checked a patient's wallet for his name and medical history, Dr. Pitkin turned to me and said, "Now you know who's in administration. They go immediately for the wallet." In a disturbingly rude resuscitative effort, an elderly lady fell down while eating dessert at a fancy restaurant. She vomited the pink mousse, and the technician cheered, "Let's get the cake out of her." Hunched over the patient with the suction device, the respiratory therapist exclaimed, "It looks as if somebody did the dishes in her mouth." During a lull in a different resuscitative effort, a technician asked what was next. He answered his own question in a dramatic theater voice: "What's the protocol saying? Pulse? Blood pressure?" These jokes express the staff's frustration, and often also anger, over carrying out futile reviving efforts.[31] I never overheard such jokes when the patient had a perceived high social viability.

Besides socializing and joking, staff also practice medical techniques on the socially but not yet officially dead patient. I did not observe resuscitative efforts in a teaching hospital but still noticed that paramedics in training would reintubate patients for practice. The nurse in charge would also show the paramedics in training how correctly to put the fibrillation pads on the patient's chest, wasting "crucial life-saving" seconds.[32]

How do these resuscitative efforts end? When a patient is considered socially dead, the staff seizes upon any indicator to pronounce the patient officially dead and stop the resuscitative effort. Once the patient's name is available, the secretary of the ED checks the computer system to see whether the patient is known to the hospital. The secretary orders the patient's charts, or the emergency physician calls the patient's physician and asks for a medical history. The emergency physician usually describes the resuscitative effort and asks the patient's physician whether the medical team should declare the patient deceased. If the patient's physician tells the emergency physician that the latter can declare the patient deceased, this pronouncement is made immediately.

Relatives and friends are another source of medical history. Family members are not allowed to enter the room where the resuscitation occurs but usually a social worker, chaplain, nurse, or the physician asks questions and keeps the family informed about the resuscitative efforts. In several of my observed cases, family members directly influenced termination of the reviving attempt. In one case, some family members were nurses in the same hospital. They asked to have the breathing tube removed "to let her die in peace."

In addition, the organizational context in which the resuscitative effort takes place influences the length of the reviving attempt. I observed one resuscitative effort called sooner than anticipated because a second code was on its way, and tending two patients in cardiac arrest would exhaust the ED staff. The length of a reviving attempt depended further on the reputation of the hospital, resuscitation styles of individual doctors and nurses, the time of the day (it is a bad time to die right before or at the changing of a shift),[33] and available resources.

When staff finds that a patient with low social viability has drafted an advance directive, they greet this news with relief. They need not go through the motions anymore. Normally, an advance directive needs to be verified by the physician in charge, but even when no advance directive can be found in the patient's file, the physician might still stop the reviving effort. In one case I observed, the team was not sure whether the patient actually had an advance directive or was merely planning to talk to her physician about it:

The chaplain enters and says, "The neighbor said that she has an aneurysm in her stomach area. She also said that she did not wanted to be operated on it. She was going to talk to her doctor tomorrow to discuss this." The physician asks, "Is she a no-code?" "According to the neighbor she is." "Why do we find this out after we have been working on her?" The head nurse takes the patient's file, which the department administrator brought into the room. She looks through it once and looks through it a second time, but she cannot find an advance directive. The physician takes the file, and together they check it again. No advance directive, no official document. The physician then decides to let the patient go anyway. He considers the patient hopeless unless she wants to have surgery.

In a different resuscitative effort, a physician informed his colleague about an advance directive that again determined the course of the resuscitative effort, even though the document was not available: "She has a living will but doesn't have it with her. It says no heroic measures. She complained of pain in her left side, and that was why she was visiting Dr. Kaufman." The physician in charge thanked his colleague and said, "Okay, we stop."

In order to put closure on the resuscitative effort, the staff prepares for an official declaration of death. This process usually involves two aspects. First, the physician or a nurse reviews the results of the most significant biomedical indicators, social characteristics, circumstantial indicators, and medical history. One patient had been unresponsive for at least twenty minutes; had no pulse, no blood pressure, asystole, or asystole approaching heart rhythm; had no spontaneous breathing; and had no positive reaction to the medication. The patient was diabetic, 76 years old. Heart disease ran through the family; nobody had seen him fall down; and the intravenous lines could not be established in the field. The physician also checked the arterial-blood–gas measurements and a chest X-ray and asked the resuscitative team about any reactions to the drugs. With enough negative evidence to justify declaring the patient legally dead, the physician pronounced this patient deceased.

The second aspect has to do with a possible cause. Declaring a patient dead does not require a cause, but most physicians prefer to know with some clinical certainty what has caused the patient's death. The physician who can point to a likely cause based on the medical history usually shares it with the staff. For example, "Because of her coronary problems, she must have had an MI [myocardial infarction]." Or "It's probably a cerebral aneurysm." If no cause is obvious, the physician or team refers to the previously gathered circumstantial information and the resuscitative effort itself. Whatever the cause, the time passed has made the difference between life and death.

The physician usually announces the patient's fate with a variation of the following phrases: "OK guys, let's call it," "I declare him dead," "We did enough. She's dead," or "You may stop." This final moment, when information crystallizes in an explicit announcement, changes the work of the emergency team. Shortly after the declaration, all resuscitative activities stop. The staff directs attention to preparing the body and cleaning the room. The nurse or house officer responsible for taking notes records the time; the respiratory therapists unhook the reservoir with which they had ventilated the patient; the nurses remove the intravenous lines; and the technician who administered the chest compressions collects the patient's clothes and jewelry for the family. The respiratory therapists, phlebologist, X-ray technicians, and physician disperse. The nurses clean the room, remove drug wrappers, and scrub away the patient's blood. The physician informs the family, accompanied by a chaplain or social worker, and fills out the patient charts. Housekeeping services clean the floor, and the technicians refill the kits with emergency drugs. When relatives are confronted with the news that their loved one has died, they often have the option of greeting the body. The staff also informs relatives that sudden death in the ED means that the coroner will look at the body. The staff inquires whether the relatives and friends would like their loved one to become an organ donor, their preference for a funeral home, and the phone numbers of immediate family.

During the majority of resuscitative efforts, the staff does not really intend to save lives. The patient's perceived low social viability combined with weak or nonexistent clinical parameters and the questionable circumstances of the cardiac arrest makes the staff feel defeated in advance. Few staff members find coping with these reviving attempts emotionally difficult. Many explained to me that they were doing patients a favor by not trying to save them. If such an assessment were based mainly on the patient's perceived social viability, the staff might condemn some patients to a premature biological death. Social death might thus become a self-fulfilling prophecy for biological death.

The legal protections to guarantee universal lifesaving care thus do not create qualitatively enhanced lifesaving; instead, they create new criteria that need to be met before a patient is pronounced dead. In Sudnow's study, once patients with presumed low social viability showed obvious signs of biological death, the staff would quickly pronounce them officially deceased. Now, a significant proportion of patients with assumed low social viability are already biologically dead when they are wheeled in the ED. The time required to exhaust the resuscitation protocols creates a new temporal interval, with legal death as the end point. This change is significant, but it does not reduce social inequality. Characteristics that marginalize certain groups of patients still predict the intensity of lifesaving fervor.

Elite Death Trajectory

In some cases, the staff knows intuitively that the patient is biologically dead, but does not act upon this knowledge and keeps resuscitating in vain. For example, I observed a resuscitative effort of a seven-month-old baby boy who was found early in the morning by his parents and—according to the paramedics—already felt stiff with rigor mortis. Still, the staff spent a full half-hour trying to resuscitate the baby before finally pronouncing him dead. Only in this resuscitative trajectory is biological death considered a failure and a personal loss.

The likelihood for this trajectory depends primarily on patient characteristics. These patients have a presumed high social viability: they are relatively young, famous, or identifiable. For example, Nurse Suzanne Jones explained how her behavior changed after she recognized a patient:

> The most recent one I worked on was one of my college professors. He happened to be one of my favorites, and I didn't even realize it was him until we were into the code and somebody mentioned his name. Then I knew it was him. All of a sudden it becomes kind of personal. You seem to be really rooting for the person. Before you were just doing your job, trying to do the best you could. But then it does get personal when you are talking to them and trying to . . . you know . . . do whatever you can do to help them through.

Resuscitative efforts are initiated in sudden infant death syndrome even when the baby has no chance of survival. One paramedic who was up for recertification told me how his instructor presented him with a scenario of SIDS in which the baby had obviously been dead for at least a couple of hours when the paramedics arrived. When the paramedic hesitated about whether he would begin a resuscitative effort, the instructor interrupted angrily, "Mike, in a SIDS case you ALWAYS resuscitate. Even if the baby is stiff as a board." SIDS is a situation in which the existential questions are undescribably painful and in which the new parents experience death as cruelly unfair. Because most babies are found in the morning by their parents and might have passed away during the night, not much can be done to revive them. Still, the ritualistic aspects of resuscitation help to make sense of a senseless death.

When confronted with a patient having a presumed high social viability, the staff goes all out to reverse the dying process. In a normal resuscitative effort, five to eight staff members are involved. In the effort to revive a nine-month-old baby, however, I counted twenty-three health-care providers in the room at one point. Specialists from different hospital services were summoned. In describing another case, Dr. Martine Chau explained the effort for one patient she identified with: "I even called the cardiologist; I very seldom do call the cardiologist on the scene, and I called him and asked him, 'Is there anything else we can do?'" In those cases, staff members do not draw each other's attention to the signs of biological death but instead focus on doing everything possible within the guidelines of the protocol. Often the physician establishes a central IV line in the patient's neck, and the respiratory therapist checks and rechecks the tube to make sure the lungs are indeed inflated. These tasks are part of the protocol but are not always performed as diligently in resuscitative attempts that follow other trajectories.

The physician might even be willing to go beyond the protocol to save the patient. For example, at the time of my observations, the number of sodium bicarbonates that could be administered was limited, and often the paramedics had exhausted the quota en route to the hospital. The physician is supposed to order more sodium bicarbonate only if the results of lab tests of blood-gas levels warrant it. In the frenzy of resuscitating a patient known to all the staff, the physician boasted to his colleague: "So much for ACLS guidelines. I gave more bicarb, and even before the blood gases were back." When a staff member's husband was the patient, nurses and physicians went out of their way to obtain a bed in intensive care.

How does such a resuscitative effort end? In contrast with the other reviving attempts, I never saw a physician make a unilateral decision. The decision to stop resuscitating a presumed valuable patient became instead a joint decision. The physician went over all the drugs that have been given, provided some medical history, mentioned the time that had elapsed since the patient collapsed, and then turned to the team and asked, "Does anybody have any suggestions?" or "I think we did everything we could. Also, Dr. Chang agrees; I think we can stop it."

For patients with a perceived high social viability, especially small children, the staff was usually sensitive to the needs of grieving relatives and friends. The effort for a five-month-old infant declared dead in the ED illustrates the staff's special response:

> Dr. Hendrickson and Linda Hibbard, a nurse, inform the relatives, while I help clean up the room. A little later, the family wants to see the baby. They enter with three people: mother, father, and grandfather. The chaplain, Rev. Ardener, comes along. When the mother sees the baby on the big stretcher, she picks him up and holds him against her face. She cries and talks to her son. She turns to us and asks, "Can I play a little game with him to say goodbye?" We nod. She sings a song to the baby. The grandfather leaves. Rivers (a nurse) follows him, crying.
>
> Rev. Ardener asks softly, "Do you want me to say a prayer?" He hesitates and adds, "We could say it together." The father bites his lip, nods, and agrees, "Good idea." The mother puts the baby back on the stretcher. Father, mother, and the chaplain hold one another by the shoulder, a little triangle of arms and bowed heads. The chaplain prays. He talks about the short life of the child and about being received in the glory of God. After the prayer the father shakes his head. He curses, "Damn, damn, damn." The mother repeats, "It is not fair. I don't want to leave my baby." She again picks the baby up and holds him to her face. She whispers, "I love you. You're a good boy." She asks, "Is it okay to hold the baby? I have never seen anybody do this before." Hibbard reassures, "It is very good to hold the baby." The father holds the baby, and the baby sighs a couple of times. This is very awkward because it feels as if the baby is gasping for air. Hibbard quickly points out that it is just sighing. "He had some air in the lungs that came out." The mother starts to cry again, "For a moment I thought he was breathing again." The mother leaves, and the father holds the baby. He then puts him down and asks, "Was there any reaction in the ambulance or here?" Hibbard shakes her head and says, "We had many

people from other departments coming over, but nobody could do anything." She adds, "It wasn't in our hands anymore." Then the father replies, "It is so difficult to leave him behind and never see him again anymore." Hibbard nods. She gives a hug, and together they leave. I walk out and see a police officer waiting in the hallway. Hibbard talks to him. While passing, I hear her say that this is a real SIDS. The baby has a long history in the hospital.

Here staff members tried to meet the relatives' spiritual and emotional needs and grieved together with the parents, giving them the opportunity to say farewell, to pray, and to ask questions about the reviving attempt. A staff member also intervened when a police officer inquired about the possibility of child abuse.[34]

I did not observe resuscitative attempts of familiar people or young patients with advance directives, but during lifesaving attempts for these patients with a presumed high social viability I never heard a staff member even suggest the possibility that the patient might have a do-not-resuscitate order. To explore this question further, I asked health-care providers how they would react when a person younger than 45, who appeared to have a chance at viability, came in with an advance directive. Staff members were torn by this dilemma and started to answer by evading the question. Most doubted that a physician would co-sign an advance directive for a young person, and others noted the variations in advance directives (ranging from no CPR to no heroic measures). Although they admitted that in principle one should always follow the wishes of a patient, they doubted that they would stop a resuscitative effort for a young person if the document were not present during the reviving attempt. When I described one of my students, a 22-year-old woman who did not want to be resuscitated, staff doubted that they would honor such a request. Nurse Ruth Berns explained,

> There are too many variables. A 22-year-old female is not supposed to have heart disease or risks. So in her case, we would ask, "Did she drown, or was she electrocuted or poisoned?" These are all things that you can treat, get rid off, and have a successful resuscitation. That 22-year-old would probably find it difficult to find a lawyer or doctor to write a statement like that. Because to me, that is the same as stating suicide in a passive-aggressive kind of way.

Several respondents added stories of patients who were saved when the staff disregarded their advance directives. A nurse supervisor prided herself on going against the wishes of a patient and his relatives, even though the patient still thought after regaining consciousness that they should not have revived him. A survey of emergency physicians found that 42 percent did not stop a resuscitative effort when an advance directive instructed them to do so.[35]

In the legal death trajectory, health-care workers are rubber-stamping the dying process. In the elite death trajectory, lifesaving measures are aggressive, hectic, and emotionally draining. But in both trajectories, the patient's perceived social viability interacts with legal requirements and clinical signs of life. Patients who are socially viable receive the most extensive effort in the ED.

Temporary Stabilization Trajectory

The temporary stabilization trajectory occurs with patients who have either a presumed high or presumed low social viability. These patients recover from cardiac arrest, but staff members doubt their own actions. Staff typically expect that the patient will suffer from a new cardiac arrest, that the patient is on a slow-dying trajectory, or that the patient will be left with limited cognitive function. For example, when a female patient was stabilized and the resuscitation team had dispersed, I was left in the room with Nurse Carolyn Lanker and the respiratory therapist Dave Johnson. Lanker asked for advice:

> Lanker: "What do you think, folks?"
> Johnson: "She is not perfusing very good, if she is perfusing."
> Lanker: "She must not even have a 60 [heart rate]."
> Johnson: "Well, I feel a carotid [pulse]. So it should at least be a 60."
> Lanker (checking the monitor): "The rate is 47."

> They talk about getting the patient a room, but the nurse doesn't think it will be necessary. "She probably is going down slowly." Lanker looks at the twelve-lead EKG and speculates, "She probably had a big MI and is now slowly going lower and lower." Her hypothesis seems to be correct, because the heart rate goes down from 47 to 46, and then one by one to 39.

I observed one resuscitative effort in which a patient was resuscitated three times in the span of a couple hours. After the first stabilization, the patient went back into cardiac arrest when X-ray technicians lifted her to take a chest X-ray. During the next resuscitative effort, all of the nursing staff and most of the attending physicians were very pessimistic about their chances of reversing the dying process. They whispered statements such as, "At a certain point, our services don't help anymore" and "Anyone wants to continue CPR? I don't think I do." A pulmonologist from outside the ED, however, insisted that they continue the lifesaving endeavor. Although the patient was eventually transferred to the intensive-care unit, staff members felt that they had performed a disservice to the patient. I could not determine whether these feelings originated from the drawn-out resuscitative effort, the patient's young age, or possible mistakes.

Patients in this situation often have presented indicators during the pre-hospital resuscitative effort that leave enough uncertainty to prevent the team from giving up right away. Often, some time had elapsed before the paramedics reached the patients, but when the paramedics arrived the patient still had a pulse. Or CPR might have been administered without defibrillation and drug therapy, but was still done expertly. These signs open a small window of opportunity to revive the patient. Even so, if the patient does not react strongly and quickly in the ED, the staff is pessimistic about lasting biological viability. The course of these resuscitative efforts often resembles a roller-coaster: the patient repeatedly gains and loses a pulse or blood pressure. The staff then wonders whether drugs are creating the signs of life and views a turn for the worse as a confirmation of the expected trajectory.

The staff reasons that when the patient does not recover immediately, a significant underlying medical problem probably can explain the downward trajectory. Healthy people do not just suffer from cardiac arrest. The resuscitation for the one person in my research who walked out of the hospital shows this reasoning. Although Marie Rivers, the nurse in charge, noted some signs of life, she expected that the patient would not last very long.[36]

> Rivers says, "We shocked him four times. He doesn't have anything left. He probably had an MI. His body is closing down."
> Dr. Nibras Nzingha agrees and refers to previous information in which the chaplain had told them that the patient had com-

plained about pain in the chest: "He probably had chest pain and didn't tell his wife about it. Well, he has good supraventricular beats." Rivers answers, "He is a mess, cardiac-wise." Nzingha adds, "The medication alone could do it [supraventricular heart beats]." He looks at the twelve-lead electrocardiogram (EKG) and says, "Well, it is rather abnormal. I cannot make anything out of it." The EKG technician asks, "Surprised?" Nzingha laughs and says, "No, I guess."

Here and in comparable cases, the events preceding the arrival in the ED, the course of the resuscitative effort, and a speculated medical history all cause the staff to remain pessimistic about the survival chances for a stabilized patient. As a result, staff members treat these patients as if they are going to die soon.

Because such patients are temporarily stabilized, the next step is to get them out of the ED and into the intensive-care unit. Yet I observed several resuscitative efforts in which the patient's condition was too precarious to warrant this transfer. For example, "The patient regains a weak faint pulse. Nurse Gerald May tries to get a blood pressure but does not succeed. The monitor shows a regularly curving rhythm. The physician wonders aloud, 'I don't think we need to call ICU. I don't trust this rhythm.'"

When the patient is precariously stabilized in the ED, the health-care providers are reluctant to ask for a transfer because they fear that the patient will code again before or during the transfer. I observed one resuscitative effort in which the patient was stabilized and later had a new cardiac arrest. This time, the staff decided not to interfere anymore, and the patient was pronounced dead.

A special complication occurs when people who seem to have a chance for survival have previously written advance directives. In most situations, information about the advance directive is apparent only well into the lifesaving attempt. In one resuscitative effort, the nursing home faxed the advance directive, but only after the patient had been more or less stabilized. Another posed ambiguity about an advance directive and illustrated the subtle message that these orders convey. The patient's EKG rhythm showed ventricular fibrillation, the medical indication for electric defibrillation. Yet because of the possibility of an advance directive, the team tried to get the patient through without defibrillating. Team members, however, remained skeptical that they could do a lot for him. Once a patient is delicately stabilized, learning of an advance directive generally fuels the staff's doubts about the patient's viability. Ironically, a living will or an advance directive becomes in itself an indication of a life-threatening condition, as staff assume that healthy people would not want to sign such a document.

At first sight, the perceived social viability of the patient does not seem overwhelmingly to affect the temporary stabilization trajectory. This trajectory is mostly a result of favorable clinical parameters and the circumstances of cardiac arrest. Yet the patient's social viability plays a crucial but indirect role. Under the staff's reluctance to revive patients who deviate from the ideal resuscitative scenario, is the fear that the resuscitated patient would have suffered brain damage. According to the dominant resuscitation theory, irreversible brain damage occurs after less than five minutes of oxygen deprivation. The staff is concerned that a patient revived after this critical period might join the ranks of a group with perceived low social viability; the severely neurologically or physically disabled. As Dr. John Cole explained to me, "There have been situations where after a prolonged down patient, we get a pulse back. My first feeling is, 'My God, what have I done?' It is a horrible feeling because you know that patient will be put in the unit and ultimately their chances of any successful walking out of the hospital without any neurological deficits are almost zero."

Physician Trevor Hendrickson described the scenario to be avoided, a resuscitative effort in which an adult survived in a vegetative state:

Physician: I remember there was a man who was having just an MRI scan done, and while he was in the machine, he had a cardiac arrest for who knows what reason. And they brought him to the ER, and we started to resuscitate him, and as we did, it looked obvious that he probably wasn't going to survive. And we gave him what we call high-dose epinephrine, and with that high dose he actually returned to a normal heart rhythm. Unfortunately, he had too much inadequate blood supply to his brain, so he ended up having not too much cognitive function.... I guess I remember that because I thought he was going to die, and I gave him a little more medicine, and he didn't. And I have always wondered whether that was the right thing to do or not.

ST: Do you think you did the right thing?

Physician: Well, in retrospect, I don't think that I did. The man is alive, but his brain is not alive, so he really is not the same person he was before. I think that from the family's point of view, they probably would have had an easier time dealing with the fact that he was dead and sort of would have gone out of their system instead of in the state he is in right now.

The patient who survives in a "vegetative" state continuously requires emotional and financial resources of relatives. Health-care providers generally consider this the ultimate "nightmare scenario," an outcome that will haunt them for years to come.[37]

With those "excesses" in mind, several of my respondents made arguments in favor of passive euthanasia. One nurse stated that she felt that in many cases attempting to resuscitate patients meant "prolonging their suffering." A technician asserted that "with [patients who have] an extensive medical history, it is inhumane to try." Another technician reflected, "Sometimes you wonder if it is really for the benefit of the patient." A chaplain even made a case for suicide (or euthanasia, depending on who is meant by the "them" in his sentence): "I feel a bit of relief knowing that if a person couldn't be resuscitated to a productive life, that it is probably just as well to have them have the right to end life." The principle that guided the rescuer's work is that a quick death is preferable to a lingering death with limited cognitive functioning. Nurse Ruth Berns said so explicitly: "The child survived with maximum brain injury and has become now, instead of a child that they [the parents] can mourn and put in the ground, a child that they mourn for years."

I found implicit in both interviews and observations a view that physically and neurologically disabled lives are difficult lives—often not worth living. Drawing from the dominant resuscitation theory, rescuers believe that the prospect of long-term physical, but particularly mental, disability is reason enough to slow a lifesaving attempt. In an age of rights for those living with disabilities and calls for the legalization of physician-assisted suicide or euthanasia, resuscitation practice indicates that health-care providers are more attuned to the physician-assisted suicide argument. People with disabilities are associated with perpetual dependence and helplessness.[38] Disability symbolizes a lack of control over life, and health-care providers fall back on the outcome over which they have the most control. Long-term disability seems to most staff members worse than biological death. In a survey of 105 experienced emergency–health-care providers (doctors, nurses, EMTs), 82 percent preferred to be dead to living with severe neurological disability.[39]

Stabilization Trajectory

Only a minority of patients stabilize after resuscitation has been initiated in the field and the paramedics have transported the patient to the ED. Stabilization is the ideal outcome for the staff, patient, and relatives, but it occurs rarely in the ED. I saw it only when circumstances were exceptionally fortunate: the patient was young or middle aged; a professional had started CPR immediately; the paramedics' response time and the transportation time were very short. These patients were not deemed either socially or biologically dead and usually had already been revived when they arrived in the ED. The nurse in charge would prepare the department for a potentially long code and request extra help from other wards or from the nurses on call at home. Often, more specialized services such as X-ray and twelve-lead EKG teams were paged and asked to wait outside to perform their technical tasks. Stabilization was also more common when the cardiac arrest occurred in the ED while the patient was being monitored: an alarm went off because the patient's heart was fibrillating, and the staff was able immediately to reverse the arrest with massage or defibrillatory shock. These episodes happened very fast, and the life-threatening crisis was over in a couple of minutes.

The stabilization trajectory involves a similar chaotic process of information gathering, centralizing, and sharing when the patient arrives. The medical staff focuses strictly on the screen of the EKG monitor. A less favorable heart rhythm quickly redefines the patient; a good heart rhythm is an impetus to search the pulse points. When a pulse is found, the heart compressions are halted; otherwise, the heart compressions continue and the technician is reminded to give deep compressions. Whereas in less viable cases, an exhausted technician might remove one hand and perform CPR single-handed, this practice is never allowed for patients with a favorable margin of viability. Because in most cases important time has already been lost in reaching the ED, the patient needs to respond quickly to ACLS.

An operational definition of viability is almost uniquely based on current biomedical readings and consists of a list of medications and tests to obtain more in-depth indicators of the patient's condition. For a patient in a dying trajectory, chest X-rays, twelve-lead EKGs, and blood gases serve as one more confirmation of the patient's condition. For a patient who might recover, these services performed soon after the patient arrives in the ED help map the needed care.

The physician decides that the patient is stabilized after cardiac function is adequately restored, but the physician does not leave the side of the patient to inform the family. One nurse constantly monitors changes in the patient's condition. Because the patient is intubated, a respiratory therapist continues manual ventilation until an automatic ventilator is connected. The physician looks for a cause of the cardiac arrest to determine which specialist should be called. The next step is to transfer the patient to an intensive-care unit. The medical staff prefers to do this as soon as possible because the patient takes up nursing time and may always backslide. Usually relatives and friends have had the opportunity to visit the patient before the transfer. In an example of such a trajectory,

> The patient was a resident in a nursing home. He collapsed while eating breakfast. The nursing-home personnel immediately laid him on the floor, and when they could not find a pulse, they called 911 and started CPR. When the paramedics arrived, they found the patient in V-fib. They shocked the patient at 200 joules, and the patient regained a pulse but was not breathing on his own. The patient was then transported to the ED. On arrival, he was unresponsive, but when the staff put a needle in his arm, he expressed pain. His pupils remained "sluggish." The physician ordered a twelve-lead EKG, a portable X-ray, and a CT scan. The EKG ruled out a myocardial infarction. After twenty-five minutes in the ED, the patient was transferred to the intensive-care unit.

I did not observe many stabilizations and am therefore reluctant to describe more detailed trajectories. Health-care workers' reports, however, indicate that so-called miracle trajectories are extremely rare. The patient may backslide and recover or backslide and be redefined to a dying trajectory, but cases in which a patient recovered after a prolonged period of unresponsiveness were uncommon.[40]

Although I did not observe advance directives in this scenario, I suspect that the staff would treat such documents as they do during the elite trajectory. Because these patients have a chance for survival, staff will probably disregard the patient's personal wishes. Health-care

providers are willing to accept a living will only when the patient ful-
fills their criteria for having one. These patients are seriously ill or old,
and staff members believe that the patient's quality of life has suffered.
Nurse Judith Kaufert explained:

> I think if a person has made very clear their wishes beforehand
> . . . especially in light of a terminal illness, a cancer, or an awful
> respiratory disease—they know that they don't have long to
> live, and the quality of their life is not very good—then it is very
> appropriate for these people to make their statements when they
> have a free mind and are conscious that they don't wish to have
> resuscitations started.

According to this nurse, the staff should always evaluate whether it is
appropriate that a patient had an advance directive.

Advance directives therefore have failed to empower patients in sudden cardiac arrest. Under the guise of increasing patient autonomy, the
documents have had the opposite result—medical paternalism. Unavailable advance directives shorten the course of resuscitative efforts
for patients already considered socially dead. At the same time, staff explained to me, the advance directives of patients considered socially viable would probably not be followed. Health-care providers follow the
wishes set forth in the advance directive when these guidelines match
their own assessment of the patient's social viability. The document
does not supersede their professional judgment.[41]

SOCIAL INEQUALITY OF SUDDEN DEATH

In most situations, the ED staff works like Charon, the ancient Roman
god who guards the entrance to the underworld. They divide the groups
of waiting souls into those who can be revived and those who cannot.
Their judgments are based on the perceived social viability of the patient, clinical parameters, and the circumstances of the cardiac arrest.
Even when staff members resuscitate aggressively, their work is not
what medical policymakers and legislators who constructed the emergency infrastructure intended. The staff reappropriate advance directives, legal imperatives to resuscitate, and biomedical protocols on the
basis of patient's presumed social viability; at the same time, the patient's social status at the end of life receives a new meaning in light of
the resuscitation apparatus.

From the staff's perspective, reaching a decision about life or death is not a great concern. Most health-care providers believe that a patient's biological fate is usually sealed before he or she reaches the ED. Different health-care providers noted that "dead is dead." They back such beliefs with the prevailing resuscitation theory, which argues that irreversible brain damage occurs after only four to six minutes of oxygen deprivation. Because the patient is deemed biologically dead anyway, the staff does not become emotionally involved in the resuscitation effort. The jocularity and casual conversations during the reviving effort betray a distanced attitude. As staff goes through the motions, a sense of urgency of life-or-death drama is absent. Dr. Hendrickson summarized the typical reasoning: "In a better world, they [the patients] wouldn't be there because there is nothing natural or sanctimonious about being declared dead in a resuscitation. It is far more natural to be declared dead with your own family in your own home."

The staff's main prerogative is to find the adequate level of care for each individual patient. This task usually means deciding that enough has been enough. Although they agree that in most cases the patients' outcomes were written in stone before they reached the ED, staff members acknowledge that with CPR and ACLS they have a slim but distinct possibility of influencing the dying process. This influence, however, is not always for the better. Concern about neurologic disability not death, is the outcome most dreaded. The staff is more concerned with protecting the patient from this potential "monstrous" outcome than with bringing people back to life. They have thus reversed the intentions of the designers of the resuscitation infrastructure.

Health-care providers are not, however, consistent in their efforts to protect patients from the potentially negative effects of the resuscitation technology. In general, the staff will not try to revive a patient unless particular characteristics render that patient socially valuable and therefore worth treating. This is the problem. The staff withholds potentially beneficial treatment because of moral judgments. The result is that the people with a perceived low social viability might die a premature biological death while patients with a perceived high social viability are resuscitated even when the effort is not indicated. Passive euthanasia for some and unnecessarily prolonged resuscitation for many is the unintended consequence of universal resuscitation techniques. Indeed, as Bauman noted, "All too often, and certainly much too often for moral comfort and political placidity, the audacious dream of killing death turns into the practice of killing people."[42] These findings are discouraging because, since Sudnow's study of sudden death in the sixties, the legislative and biomedical initiatives have failed to diminish the rampant social rationing during resuscitative efforts. In a new technical and social configuration, who one is still determines how and whether one will die.

Instead of concluding that social inequality is an inevitable part of resuscitating, the scientific and legislative initiatives might not have addressed the broader societal foundations of social inequality. Unfortunately, the attitudes of the emergency staff reflect and perpetuate those of a society poorly equipped, culturally and structurally, to accept the elderly, seriously ill, and disabled as people whose lives are valued and valuable.[43] As the need for an Americans with Disabilities Act shows, those with disabilities or serious illness are considered socially dead not only in the ED but also in the outside world.[44] The staff has internalized beliefs about the presumed low worth of elderly and disabled people to the extent that more than 80 percent would rather be dead than live with a severe neurological disability. As gatekeepers between life and death, they have the opportunity explicitly to execute the subtle but pervasive moral code of the wider society. Just as schools, restaurants, and modes of transportation became the battlegrounds and symbols in the civil-rights struggle, medical interventions such as genetic counseling, euthanasia, and resuscitative efforts represent the sites of contention in the disability- and elderly-rights movement.[45] At the same time, the staff's actions also reflect the widespread disenchantment with unnecessary prolonging of life. Terminating unnecessary medical interventions during the dying process receives much public-opinion support. Resuscitators in the ED try to reconcile emotionally charged opposing value claims while managing patient trajectories.

Rationalizing medical practice and providing legal accountability have only accentuated social inequality. Biomedical protocols have become part of the problem because the staff relies on those theories to justify limiting resuscitation for people who might become disabled. The "chain of survival" theory has become the major framework for "walking" ineffective codes. Legal initiatives mostly stimulated the predominance of resuscitative efforts at the expense of other ways of dying and have been unable to protect marginalized groups. The staff is legally obligated to go through lengthier resuscitative motions with more patients, but the staff need not want to revive those patients. The widespread adoption of CPR has changed resuscitating in the ED, but it has not erased social inequality; it has displaced and imbued it with new legal and medical practices. It might be more fruitful to reverse the momentum of the legal initiatives and instead guarantee that only those for whom lifesaving is indicated will receive resuscitative care.

In the blurry space between worthwhile lives and proper deaths, resuscitative efforts in the ED reflect submerged and subtle attitudes of the wider society. The ED staff enforce and perpetuate our refusal to let go of life and to accommodate certain groups. But because health-care providers implement our moral codes, they are the actors who might be able to provide new perspectives. Even with the rampant social rationing, staff members seem to differ from the wider society in their views of death and dying. They are willing to let go of life and not to revive when others hesitate to do so. In the next chapter, I will explain how these attitudes about death evolve during the career of a health-care provider and how they might open avenues for more profound changes in resuscitating.

6 "There Is a Code and a Code"

> We get a lot of them [resuscitative efforts]. Everyone gets all excited
> because there is a code coming in. I don't. Because I know—there is
> a code and a code—there are some that you know are going to be
> pronounced in a matter of minutes and then there are some that we
> got quick enough and this is going to be a real strong effort.
> (Nurse Carolyn Lanker)

THE ROUTINES OF EMERGENCIES

RESUSCITATIVE EFFORTS are emergencies for relatives and patients, and routines for medical professionals.[1] The casual conversations during compressions and ventilations, the laid-back attitude of some health professionals, and the ease with which a resuscitative attempt is incorporated into the daily schedule and forgotten afterwards implies that most lifesaving efforts are routine work. The staff rarely become overwhelmed by the life-or-death situation. Still, not all resuscitative efforts in emergency departments are routine for the staff. In some cases and for some health-care providers, resuscitative efforts require extra adjustments, sometimes institutional and technical, but mostly psychosocial under the form of debriefing or counseling. In those situations, the resuscitative effort is also an emergency.

Viewed in the context of our society's general refusal to face sudden death, resuscitative efforts are an amazing routine. Even if the health-care provider's decision making remains profoundly ethically problematic, ED professionals can reach decisions about life and death. In every resuscitative effort, they are the first persons to say that enough is enough and that we should accept that death has occurred. The decisions that others dread to make are their bread and butter. Health-care providers seem to possess an acceptance about the terminality of life fostered by years of experience that the rest of us do not have. Their professional familiarity with intervening between life and death has demystified death and dying to the extent that these processes become part of their jobs. How do resuscitative efforts—and by implication, death and dying—become routine for ED workers, and under which circumstances do they remain emergencies?

We can glimpse a coping mechanism to deal with sudden death when Carolyn Lanker, a nurse with twenty-seven years of experience in emergency medicine, states, "There is a code and a code." Not every "code," or resuscitative effort, is the same, and not every attempt is worthy of the label "resuscitation" for each person involved. According to Lanker, there are at least two very different kinds of resuscitative attempts:

> The first category is unnecessary. It is a worthless effort often times. I see it as degrading the dignity of the person. I feel that we are spending unnecessary money for things that are never going to change, and I think that I have a lot of reservations in accepting and treating all the codes that come in. The second category [is] if it is a witnessed arrest, a drowning, a shock, something that is tragic—just sudden deaths—and somebody is there right away, then you have a chance. You really, really get involved in it, and want to see it come to a good ending.

The first situation is not really experienced as a resuscitative endeavor. The other gets her adrenaline going. The latter retains the character of an emergency. The former is part of a routine. It is likely that Lanker becomes emotionally involved only with the second category. She clearly expresses her reservations about the necessity and effectiveness of the first category of lifesaving attempts. Categorizing a resuscitative effort helps Lanker develop a perspective on the lifesaving.

For the outsider or neophyte in the field, all resuscitative efforts look the same. It is one hectic rush in which a group of people does a variety of things to a dying person. The experienced health-care provider, however, can distinguish among a wide variety of codes and make sense of the resuscitative effort by putting it in a subcategory. The emergency staff worker knows what can be expected and is able to anticipate the flow of events on the basis of the kind of code. Because of this process, the worker comes to accept the finality of life.[2]

BECOMING A RESUSCITATOR

The demystification of death begins early in the career of the health-care provider. It is part of learning the tricks of the trade, of becoming a nurse, physician, chaplain, respiratory therapist, or ED technician. Not many people are mindful of this gradual process of growing awareness. It evolves over time and is difficult to track down, even through a combination of interviews and observations. Still, in moments of re-flection, my respondents offered insights into their socialization process and remembered some key events. John Delaney, a nurse with more than twenty years of experience in emergency medicine, recalled an il-lustrative incident:

> I just had a recent experience where I was talking to somebody who went through a resuscitation for the first time, and I knew they were upset about it. And when we were talking, I thought they were upset because they knew who the person was, but that wasn't it—they were upset because it wasn't the way it was in class. They had no idea. They were told how to go through the procedures, and they did that, but they weren't told what else to expect. So they didn't expect anything else. And then when the guy was there, and all these things were going on, there were things they were never even told about, that they never even thought about, and I think the inference is that if you do everything right, then things are going to work out.

In conversation, Delaney assumed that the novice was distressed be-cause he knew the patient. Such recognition is one of the key features of a tragic resuscitative effort. The neophyte was upset, however, be-cause the resuscitative effort did not produce the expected result. In schools and training sessions, CPR and ACLS are taught as pre-struc-tured medical techniques. If you follow a certain algorithm, make sure to give particular drugs, artificially ventilate, and continue closed-chest compressions in the right sequences, the resuscitation will work out. Those procedures are practiced over and over again on the mannequin "Resusci-Anne,"[3] and, as Ginny Kincaid, a respiratory therapist, re-marked ironically, "Anne is always OK. She never looks blue. She never vomits." The educational system and media focus on resuscitating as the correct performance of a technique gives the novice health-care provider—like the general public—the overall impression that once you start CPR, you can expect an outcome in which the patient survives.

In the ED, the novice quickly learns that procedures and protocols are only part of a resuscitative effort. Everett Hughes called this the "re-ality shock."[4] Several respondents mentioned the "awakening" after their first real resuscitative effort. Mark Lanchester, a nurse who had worked as an ED technician, recalled how he broke the ribs of the first patient he resuscitated:

ST: Could you give me an outstanding example of a resuscitative effort?

ML: The very first, the first thing that I can remember is my first cardiac arrest as an EMT after my CPR training. The thing that really strikes me most there was that when I did CPR, ribs cracked. And no one ever told me that. Even during my CPR training, no one ever said, "When you are pushing on the sternum, you are going to break ribs, especially in older people. It is going to happen; expect it." No one ever told me that. So when I first did CPR, I heard the ribs crack, felt the ribs crack. The patient didn't make it. I felt that it was my fault. I thought that I had broken a rib and punctured a lung, punctured the heart, and therefore they never came back. I have since learned that that wasn't true, but that one sticks out highly.

ST: How did you learn it wasn't your fault?

ML: I sat there, and I did everything that we were supposed to do during a [cardiac] arrest. Then the doctor called it, and that relieved us of our duties . . . and at that time I was just an EMT, so our duties were just to do CPR. And I left. I left. I went alone. I went back up to the ambulance, and I kicked the ambulance tires, I was so mad, I was so frustrated. . . . I had done this. That went on for about an hour. And then one of my co-workers came up to me and sat down and talked with me and explained that that was what had happened. And it made it better. It made it better, but at first it [felt like it] was my fault.

Similarly, a nurse manager told me how recovery-room staff keep a code book of first code experiences for all the nurses on the ward. When they have a new nurse come in and she or he goes through a first resuscitative effort, they present the code book and show the stories. The narratives function as a written memory of the uncertainty and the fumbles. Sharing them is a form of encouragement and reflection. The stories also serve as a reminder that, although rare, resuscitative attempts happen on the recovery ward, and one should always be prepared.

For others, the epiphanic insight that resuscitative efforts involve more than following protocols comes after a series of resuscitative attempts.[5] Chaplain Dora Johnson explained,

In my training as a chaplain at South Hospital, we had so many resuscitations coming in, I just got to the point where if I had to stand there and watch them pumping on another person, I just didn't think I could do it. And I had to mentally get beyond that. I had to see my role as what it really was. I couldn't do anything for that person as a chaplain, but I could do something for that family. And to be there for whatever they needed—however simple or however complex or however frustrating or irate or whatever. But it was a good learning experience for me, because I think if I could have stayed with that kind of callousness, I wouldn't be able to help families today.

For the chaplain, "all pumping on the chest" seemed futile. Once she understood that family members have different needs, her position in the resuscitative effort became more apparent.

Reflecting on actions, accumulated experience, changes in CPR protocols,[6] and guidance from colleagues teaches the health-care provider that resuscitative efforts are not always about saving lives. Joan Stelling and Rue Bucher [7] label this the acquisition of a "vocabulary of realism." Nurse Gerald May reflected, "When I first went down to the emergency room, I had so many patients in cardiac arrest that never lived that I really came to the realization that most of them aren't really going to." A student nurse added, "I was kind of surprised because I think we have all been brainwashed to believe that they are saving all these people, but really we are not saving many people." Every real-life resuscitative effort articulates and challenges some of the preconceptions and initial expectations.[8] And instead of depending on simulations with a mannequin or textbook protocols, the health-care provider relies on a growing set of personalized experiences shared with others and made part of an emergency department subculture. As Nurse Ruth Berns recalled, "In the beginning you think you can save everyone; this is what they teach you. But then it takes you a long time before you actually save somebody. I remember after about two, three years in the ER when I had my first save, thinking, 'Oh, this does work after all.'" Similarly, Josh Brittan, the ED technician, recalled his early CPR days in military service:

Well, when I worked for a local ambulance service here, we used to have a club. We called it the "CPR club." You were a member of the club as long as you were zero for something. What I mean by zero for something is that every time you did

CPR on a patient, you marked it down as one. If a person died you were zero for one, zero for two, zero for three. Before I had actually seen CPR done in the civilian life, I was zero for twelve. Then I got out of the club, because I was one for thirteen.

The respiratory therapist Dave Johnson had a similar turning event later in his career:

About eight years ago, one code that stuck out in my mind was a code that I was the first responder, and it's probably only been twice in the fifteen years that I have worked here. I did mouth-to-mouth on this patient. I intubated, and we went through ACLS. The patient was defibrillated. He went to a normal-size rhythm. He went to the unit. He woke up the next day. He was extubated. The next day I talked to him. It was totally self-gratifying. I was just ecstatic. On cloud nine for about three days, until he then died.

This recognition that not all patients—in fact, few patients—are going to make it paves the way for creating different categories of lifesaving attempts. Just as becoming an ethnographic insider might consist of learning to distinguish between a wink and a mere twitch of the eye,[9] the health-care provider learns to distinguish between "a successful code" and a "bad resuscitative event."

Usually, the health-care provider encounters a resuscitative effort that leaves a big impression. For example, one ED technician told me about a resuscitative effort early in her career in which she tried to revive the grandmother of her best friend. She experienced this resuscitative effort as very dramatic and different from all the others she had done before. Other respondents told stories of taking care of terminal or dying family members, which attuned them to the importance of taking care of family members. Mark Lanchester recalled when he started questioning the impact of his actions:

[B]ut after being on so many cardiac arrests, you really begin to doubt, are we doing any good? I remember on one we did, and it was the first one I got back, the patient came back to life. Came back, and he ended up being in the hospital for three days . . . ended up with brain damage and died three months later. And I was kind of like: why? Did I do any good or not? Did I make the situation better or worse? And I can't say that I did.

Jennifer Cohen, a nurse with twenty-two years of resuscitative experience, attributed her sensitivity to the needs of family members to her own experience as one of three nurses in a family dealing with her ailing father:

> I was in this situation where I almost had to resuscitate my own father, and he passed away two years ago . . . cardiac . . . and had coded twice prior to dying. I know how it feels. I know the frustration of the family that goes through and lives with some of the heart diseases and waits for that impending time to come . . . and it is supposedly easier, because they know it is coming, but it is not.

Other health-care providers personally experienced the tragedy of still-births or SIDS, or they knew family members, friends, or colleagues who went through those events. These experiences might lead to a perspective on resuscitative efforts that has little in common with the textbook notions. For example, Jennifer Cohen admitted, "The things that stand out really don't have anything to do with the codes; it is something else." The different aspects that discern heterogeneity in seeming homogeneity accumulate over time. They progress conversation after conversation, experience after experience, resuscitative effort after resuscitative effort, gradually evolving into a set of categories. This scheme of categories is part of the culture of the ED and is shared with newcomers.[10]

Because resuscitation invokes a division of labor, members of each professional group have their own typical categorizations. For example, the task of coordinating the attempt is typical for the nurse in charge and exceptional for the ED technician. As Chapter 5 explains, nurses are well aware of the different factors that need to be balanced to reach a decision. But because the ED technician usually gives the physically exhausting chest compressions, the technician will experience the length of a resuscitation differently from a physician, who often leaves the resuscitation room to fill out forms, see other patients, or talk to relatives.

Through the blend of personal and collective experiences with dying and resuscitative efforts, the health-care providers create their own categorization scheme based on particular aspects of a resuscitative effort. These categories are not necessarily internally consistent or mutually exclusive. Some respondents mentioned all of them but did not weigh them equally. Like the resuscitative trajectories discussed in Chapter 5, patient characteristics such as age and seriousness of illness are distinguishing indicators. But where resuscitative trajectories illuminate the process of decision making, the categories developed by health-care providers refer to the meaning of a reviving attempt.

Major Categories

Most respondents distinguished three kinds of resuscitative efforts. They remembered an effort as successful, bad, or tragic. A successful resuscitative effort is one that the respondent feels good about, usually because something that the team member considers most important in resuscitations worked out. The most striking feature of a bad resuscitative effort is that the effort did not correspond to the health-care provider's expectations and caused anger, frustration, or even disgust. In a tragic resuscitative effort, the outstanding feature becomes an emotional drain on the care provider.

These three categories, however, do not cover the entire universe of resuscitative attempts. There is a fourth category—or, more precisely, non-category. In this residual category belong attempts that are not successful, bad, or tragic. In it are resuscitative efforts that are not really efforts or those so colorless that the care provider does not remember them.

The Successful Resuscitative Effort

Health-care providers distinguish between two general subcategories of successful resuscitative efforts: for some, survival is the bottom line, and success is expressed in the patient's outcome at the end of the resuscitative effort. A good outcome, however, varies widely and can be mapped on a continuum of quality of life after the resuscitative effort. The second subcategory focuses less on survival. Here, survival is a bonus, but success depends on different criteria such as following a smooth resuscitative course, supporting the family, or obeying the patient's wishes.

Survival as the Bottom Line   For several of my respondents, a successful resuscitation could be defined only in terms of its outcome. What was a "successful" outcome, however, differed across medical groups and depended on the patient's viability and quality of life. One respondent defined success negatively as "those that leave the emergency room in any other category than expired," but most specified what a good outcome would be. The different criteria for a success can be mapped

TABLE 6-1. *Categorization of Resuscitative Efforts*

Category	Characteristic
SUCCESSFUL	Outcome-dependent
	Viable rhythm
	Pulse-blood pressure
	Neurological damage
	Before = after
	Outcome-independent
	To do everything possible
	Family
	Follow wishes
BAD	Conflicts-disagreements
	Outside interference
	Mistakes and fumbles
TRAGIC	Young patient
	Famous-identifiable patient
	Boundary experience
	Beating the odds
UNCATEGORIZED	DOA
	Pulseless nonbreather
	Pulseless nonbreather

on an continuum: on one side is a viable heart rhythm, on the other is the ability to walk out of the hospital with full neurological functioning.

A few respondents defined a good outcome as "having some kind of a viable rhythm." By this, they meant the EKG rhythm, which identifies the electric activity in the heart. Viability depended on the healthcare provider's interpretation. An identifiable rhythm is the most optimistic criterion for a successful outcome because the indicator does not mean the patient has unassisted breathing capacities or any cognitive functioning left. It means only that some kind of a viable heartbeat has been established. This criterion was used only by ED technicians and nurses who had previously worked as paramedics, and they added that this measure was insufficient for their work in the ED. For paramedics, a viable rhythm is a sufficient criterion to transfer the patient to the ED staff, but in the ED, a viable rhythm means that the effort is not yet finished. The heartbeat needs to pick up and be followed by other indicators, because the rhythm might be a side effect of drugs and might quickly fade away.

The next criterion on the continuum is stabilizing the patient for transfer to the intensive-care unit. As Ken Glasser, a nurse supervisor, explained, "From my point of view, if I can get them to the intensive-care unit and they are doing okay, I can consider it successful." Respondents also suggested that the patient might be receiving any kind of response to defibrillation and drugs or might just have a pulse, blood pressure, and preferably also unassisted breathing. Dr. Nibras Nzingha was more specific: "We consider a success if we get a pulse and a [blood] pressure. Basically, it is a success if they are not dead in the emergency department."

Other criteria make an important difference between a resuscitation and a reanimation. A resuscitation consists of artificially restoring circulatory and respiratory functions. A reanimation goes further, so that not only lung and heart are restored but also the "anima," or soul (i.e., neurological functioning), is brought back. Different respondents from all professions agreed that this criterion could already be met when the patient had limited neurological damage. Dr. David Reznikov offered a subtle definition of a successful resuscitative effort: "A successful resuscitation is the patient who is discharged from the hospital with some but a reconcilable neurological deficit."

Reflecting the official outcome statistics, most respondents considered full survival the only successful outcome. One respondent put it succinctly: "The only ones that are successes are the ones that are restored with cerebral functions." Several respondents emphasized that the patient should be able to "walk" out of the hospital; others stated plainly that the person should have exactly the same quality of life before and after the resuscitative effort. Nurse Marie Rivers gave an example:

A successful resuscitative effort is someone like I saw Sunday. I saw him April 15 and then I saw him again today. April 15, when he came in, he was actively having a heart attack. We gave him the trombolitics, try to break up the clot. It wasn't working. He went up to cath lab, was still awake at that time but didn't have much of a blood pressure, and in the cath lab he coded, and they shocked him about fifty times, and then he went straight from the cath lab to open-heart surgery, I went to see him later in the cath lab, and he was still awake, and he had all his faculties. Then I saw him again Sunday and he looks great. He doesn't have any problems with thinking, walking. To me that is a successful resuscitation; it wasn't one that we did, but we started the process.

The respondents who defined success in these terms looked primarily at the patient's condition after the resuscitative effort. Marie Rivers further explained how she considered resuscitated patients who do not keep their full capacities: "They are just, I mean, they are resuscitated to the point of having a blood pressure and their heart beating. I guess just unsuccessful, they are unsuccessful but resuscitated."

Several respondents also indicated that over time they had changed their opinion of a "good outcome." Initially, they might have considered successes only the patients who could walk out of the hospital, but after a number of resuscitative efforts they expanded their definition to include people who were transferred out of the ED.

Outcome as a Bonus In the second subcategory of success, the final patient outcome is less important than the process of resuscitating, providing support to the family, or abiding by the personal wishes of the patient. Although it is in some cases better to end up with a surviving patient, success may depend on assessments different from patient outcome. Adam Dinkes, a highly regarded and experienced ED technician, replied to my question about what he considered a successful resuscitative effort: "Well, not necessarily whether the patient survives or not. Maybe I've gotten past that point." The most often cited criterion is "to do everything humanly possible." Dinkes continued, "But being that we are in a location where we are trying to teach people how to do this to the best of their ability, a successful resuscitation is that we did the best we possibly could for this person." What does the best possible mean? A smooth operation and team interaction are the main elements. Dr. Martine Chau explained: "I think a resuscitation is good when everyone functions together—like a well-oiled machine, I guess you could say."

Other respondents saw success as doing everything possible from their own perspective. If they contributed to the team as they were supposed to do, they considered the resuscitative effort successful. Shannon Meltzer, a respiratory therapist, provided this description:

From what we are taught and what our function is here, we have to bag, to ventilate the patient, and my concern is nothing else. I have to be at the head, and I have to see if that patient is intubated properly, and the tube is secured properly, and that we ventilate the patient properly. We have to make up for the lactic acidosis that occurs when they do code, so we hyperventilate them. After that, first blood-gas comes back, if I have a good PO_2 200–400 and a low CO_2 then I have done a good job. I have blown up the carbon dioxide. That is what my job is, and that is my primary job.

A third example occurs when team members do everything possible within the current state of knowledge. Dr. Chau explained: "In a resuscitation you have twenty-five different things that can happen. So if there is a patient on the table, with a full arrest, has no heartbeat at all, whatever the protocol set up by the American Heart Association demands, and whatever is right to do, I will follow those steps. And I think that is a very successful resuscitative effort."

All the instances of this criterion boils down to giving the patient the best possible chance for survival. The outcome, however, is secondary to the effort. For one ED technician, the outcome was totally irrelevant. According to him, the "positive attitude" of the team members was the only aspect that counted and made a resuscitative effort successful. If the team members had a positive attitude, they were bound to obtain the best possible outcome.

For some care providers, a surviving patient is better but frequently out of reach, and the focus is instead on the family. This perspective is less prevalent among respiratory therapists, who usually do not come into contact with family members after resuscitative efforts (but who might see stabilized patients afterward on other wards). Nurse supervisors, physicians, chaplains, and social workers were more likely to mention this aspect of a good resuscitative effort and emphasize its importance. Dr. John Cole vocalized their view:

> In matter of fact, the family becomes a resuscitation in itself. I spend much more energy. Even when I am with the patient for the sixty or ninety seconds, if that, I almost don't think about the patient, and I prepare myself for the emotional resuscitation or the emotional guidance of the family in their grief. The patient was gone before they got there.

Regardless of patient survival, some emergency medical staff tried to be attentive to the family's need for information and support. Nurse Jennifer Cohen, who had extensive personal experience with cardiac illness, provided a distinctive sensitivity:

My thoughts throughout the entire resuscitative effort, even prior to the arrival, is the family. Who is going to be with that family; who is going to support them? And that they are being notified throughout the resuscitative effort what is going on, to prepare them if it is going to be a long haul, or if things are not good and are not going to get better. I think they deserve that.

After doing everything possible and taking care of relatives, a third criterion for success independent of outcome is following the patient's wishes. Here, a resuscitative effort is successful when the team abides by the patient's wishes or by those of a family member. One nurse who previously worked on an AIDS ward recalled how they did "custom codes." Every patient could decide what was wanted or not wanted in case of a resuscitation. This determination became for him the criterion for a successful resuscitative effort in the ED.

All these categories of success focus on some aspect of the resuscitative effort apart from the outcome. It is noteworthy that in those categories death is not necessarily the enemy or grounds for failure. Dr. Jim Atkins, a young physician, admitted, "As bad as it sounds, there are many times that I feel satisfied when it was done very well; the entire resuscitative effort was done very well, very efficiently, even though the patient didn't make it."

The Bad Resuscitative Effort

The criteria for defining a successful resuscitative attempt suggest that efforts that leave patients with extensive neurological damage or those in which patients die are not automatically considered "bad." Even staff who consider a success to be only one in which the patient fully recovers also take into account the many unknowns. One can never know for certain when a patient went into cardiac arrest, and thus whether the patient will be left with neurological damage. Often, a vegetative state appears twenty-four to forty-eight hours after the patient stabilizes.

Still, resuscitation staff provided overwhelming consensus about what makes a resuscitative effort bad. Typical of a bad resuscitative effort is that rescuers feel that they are performing a disservice for the patient but are forced to continue because of an unequal power relationship among team members. A common source of bad resuscitative efforts is conflict among staff members. Although the goal is to foster a united front,[11] certain situations present conflicting definitions of viability. I observed one in which a couple of caretakers believed that the patient was still viable while the others were ready to call it quits. In one case, the team had summoned an anesthesiologist to help them intubate a baby. The anesthesiologist failed repeatedly with different tube sizes and kept murmuring that "the baby is stiff." Nurse Jennifer Cohen provided a similar example:

> This fellow that we had to resuscitate last week had a type of tumor that sends little tendrils down through the brain, and basically, it's fatal. They do some surgery to try to get as much as they can. Well, this man had a bad prognosis, and the way he went was actually a blessing. He actually threw a blood clot, and he just died instantly. I was a bit disturbed at that code that they went and worked on him for an hour and never got, never got a rhythm back at all. That's distressing. There is a point where you say, "Come on, you are going to resuscitate him so he can die this terrible agonizing death?" That is ridiculous.

The way a potential conflict resolves depends on the position of the disbeliever in the medical hierarchy. If the physician in charge believes that the patient is still viable and the rest of the staff does not, the staff has little choice but to go along. But staff members are not powerless in such reviving attempts. They will try to convince a particularly persistent physician to quit.[12] I regularly observed nurses dropping hints to physicians that there probably was not much they could do for the patient or suggesting other treatments instead. A nurse labeled this process "egging them along." This happened more often when the physician was inexperienced or from outside the ED. In one case, I noted,

> The team is becoming impatient. The head nurse asks the physician what is next. The physician goes over the list of all the medication and then orders one more epinephrine. The head nurse replies, "I think that under the circumstances we tried everything." The physician asks if there was any response at the scene. The nurse answers, "There was no response at any moment." The physician then asks to stop CPR. The head nurse asks, "Why don't you call it?" She continues, "It's 5:52." Then she writes down, "Code called." She leaves. The physician is stunned. The other nurses try not to burst out in laughter. Finally, the physician calls the patient after having felt for the pulse again.

When a nurse, technician, paramedic, or respiratory therapist is invested in the patient and thinks the person is still viable but the physician does not agree, care providers can do very little. They can admonish their colleagues to keep working, but the physician's decision prevails. One nurse administrator described her task as being "a constant reminder" to the team and readily admitted that her reminders were aimed at what she considered fair results. A colleague gave an example:

> There was a resuscitative effort not so long ago where the patient was a drug addict and we are going through the code and I say, "This guy is a known drug addict." And the doctor turns around and says smartly, "No kidding." "Well," I say, "you might want to try some [name drug]." And he said, "Oh, okay yes, that is probably a good idea."

In this case, the administrator's reminder is a subtle way to prompt the physician to a more aggressive treatment. If a different result is anticipated, the nurse in charge of the resuscitative effort might choose not to remind physicians of the next step in the protocol or—as happens regularly—might opt not to mention variations in pulse or blood pressure while the physician was out of the resuscitation room. To me, several of the younger members of the resuscitation team expressed surprise at the quickness with which some patients were "called." Paramedics who "busted their asses" to get the patient in a more or less viable rhythm into the ED were especially disappointed that "all that work was for nothing" when the patient was called shortly after their arrival. Don Clark, a paramedic, recalled such an incident:

> One patient we brought in was in and out of a viable rhythm. By the time we would get back to the hospital, he was biting the tube and breathing on his own. But when we transferred him over the bed, he went back into V-fib, and we shocked him out of it. Then they wanted to move him again, and he went back into V-fib. They called it. This could have been a different outcome if they were more aggressive, used different drugs…. It was very tough…. We talked about it for a long time.

At the same time, paramedics are often amused by the amount of work the ED staff is willing to go through to revive a patient whom they have observed in a nonviable rhythm for the past ten minutes.

Almost all respondents volunteered that resuscitative efforts that go on for too long are bad. Eleanor Banks, a respiratory therapist, provided an extreme example:

> EB: I had several bad experiences with resuscitations. One that especially sticks out in my mind was a couple of years ago. I remember there was an incident in which there was a woman in her fifties who coded in what was at that time our coronary intensive-care unit. And we proceeded to continue the code from I think it was 11:00 in the evening, and then the code continued until about 4:00 in the morning. As R[espiratory] T[herapist]s there were three of us on, and we were taking turns in that room, and that must have been the worst experience that I have had with a resuscitation. And the lady did end up dying, and it almost got to the point where it felt we were cruel to her. We were not doing her any favors.
>
> ST: Why did you continue for so long?
>
> EB: I think the physician thought that if he could give the right combination of drugs and if he could have the drugs work in her system for long enough. Although we had to shock her repeatedly, and we had her intubated, and every time she coded, we had to take her of the vent[ilator] and bag her, and she was then sort of okay for ten to fifteen minutes, he thought that he could bring her out of it. Needless to say that it didn't work. It is difficult [to say] whether it was just heroics on his part or whether he got caught up in his effort or what. It was not pleasant.
>
> ST: Was there any way to express that?
>
> EB: Yes, we expressed our feelings to him frequently, but he just said that he wanted to continue on. And since he was the physician in charge of the code, you just have to go with it. It was not a pleasant time, and I don't think that anybody walked away from this feeling very good, the physician included.

A resuscitative effort that spans five hours is exceptional. What is not so exceptional is that nurses, respiratory therapists, chaplains, and ED technicians blame the physician for stretching the resuscitative attempt beyond reason. Because physicians are in charge, it is their decision to stop the resuscitative measures,[13] but it is not always the physician who extends them. A chaplain recalled how a patient's spouse did not want to face the impending death, so her husband was resuscitated six times in a row.

Although one physician acknowledged that he sometimes saw the frustration in the nurses' eyes when he would order another round of medication, and another admitted that "nurses pull their hair out because I drag this resuscitation out for twenty more minutes," they in turn complained of outside pressures that forced them to continue many resuscitative efforts. Dr. Brian Waxman, an older physician, bitterly stated, "I go through a ritual that is designed for lawyers; that is how I feel." A different physician complained about the emergency system in which EMTs and paramedics just bring in everything and ACLS guidelines require them to run through several rounds of medication and therefore stretch the attempt unnecessarily.

The largest category of bad resuscitative efforts are those that exhaust any benefit for the patient but still continue because of external pressures. In addition, respondents also mentioned the efforts that are characterized by fumbles, mistakes, misunderstandings, shortages, or oversupply of personnel and equipment. For example, the first time I was paged was not for a resuscitative effort but for a patient who was expected to go into cardiac arrest soon. A surgeon wanted to implant a pacemaker in the ED because the operating rooms were occupied. At the last minute, the team received the news that an operating room was free after all. Quickly the patient was moved on a stretcher, with IV pumps, heart monitor, and oxygen bottles. Unbeknownst to the team, a new carpet had been laid in the hallway. In the rush, the IV pumps became stuck behind the carpet, and all IV lines were ripped out of the patient's arm.[14]

In several resuscitative efforts, the defibrillator did not work because the batteries were dead (the ACLS textbook warns, "A dead defibrillator means a dead patient.").[15] Other technical problems include a machine misfiring with a big spark because the patient's chest is wet from perspiration. In countless efforts I observed, the leads of the EKG monitor became loose, and the monitor malfunctioned. In other resuscitative attempts, not enough or too many personnel were in the room, drugs were in short supply or mixed up, no room was available, veins were impossible to find, the team members misunderstood one another, or lines of authority were unclear. The result was a compromised attempt to save the patient. In such cases, the health-care providers wondered what might have been different if things had worked better. As nurse Judith Kaufert described:

> Then there are some that came in, and maybe you weren't quite ready. Maybe you got a thirty-second notice, and they were there. Somebody had a difficult time getting the patient intubated so you couldn't get them oxygenated well. You couldn't get an IV in, save your soul, nothing went right. You didn't get the pumps that you needed to do. You didn't get the equipment to work right, and then you feel bad, because what if we were able to get him intubated? You ask yourself, "What if we could have done more?"

Nurse supervisors and respiratory therapists who work in the ED and the other floors of the hospital divulged that these "what if?" questions sometimes haunt them after resuscitative efforts in which personnel were inexperienced in resuscitating.

While most respondents singled out aspects that go wrong during reviving, Adam Dinkes, an observant technician, described the entire resuscitative effort as a disservice to the patient. His reply was the most explicit admission that resuscitative efforts can be iatrogenic (physician induced): "In fact, we can overshoot, too. We try really hard to keep everything on the median level, but we can screw up and overshoot, too. And then we can make the patient actually worse than better. We can actually maybe even not be able to resuscitate them because of what we do."

The Tragic Resuscitative Effort

The final outcome, contact with the family, the smooth flow, following the patient's wishes, or the length of the resuscitative effort are not the most salient features of tragic resuscitative attempts. Instead an outstanding, atypical patient characteristic can color the code and create a "frenzied" atmosphere for some or all of the staff members.[16] These lifesaving attempts are difficult or remarkable. While in the bad resuscitative effort, the medical professional might be frustrated with the physician or with the system, in the tragic resuscitative effort the health-care provider becomes emotionally involved with the patient or relatives. These efforts are second-guessed, extensively debriefed, and played over and over again. Which resuscitative efforts have such an impact? Tragic resuscitative efforts comprise four subcategories: very young patients, famous and identifiable patients, boundary experiences, and heroic efforts.

The age of the patient is the most outstanding feature of a tragic cardiac arrest or sudden death. As Chapter 5 explains, almost all respondents noted that resuscitating young patients was much more difficult than working on older patients.[17] Nurse Jennifer Cohen explained: "When it is adults, you can kind of detach yourself a bit because you generally don't know the person. It is different if you know the person. But pediatrics, it's very hard for me to keep that level of detachment. I think about the child's parents, what they must have thought at the last minute, or what they must be experiencing now. That is a real biggie, what their parents are going through at the moment that we are doing it." Nurse John Delaney agreed, "I don't want to get too emotionally involved with it. I do what I have to do. But when it comes to kids, I get a little bit lost in it." Even the length of a resuscitative effort is experienced differently with children. As Dr. Hendrickson described, "In more cases I probably would not have gone on as long, as far as adults are concerned. Kids, everybody just goes all out. I have never seen anybody call kids early. In most adult cases I feel that—well, not most, but a fair number of them—they go on longer than they should." The sudden end of a potentially long life create a special tragic subtext to the resuscitative effort.

This subtext is accentuated for two categories of young patients, SIDS patients and abused children. Harry Kochan, a social worker, commented, "One of the most difficult deaths in regards to resuscitation that I encountered in this environment is SIDS. Children, that is *the* most difficult population. Somewhere we have a written or unwritten rule that babies do not die. Old people die. You die from critical accidents. But you don't die when you are a baby. You have your whole life ahead of you. And that is hard for the staff." SIDS children are difficult exactly because in true SIDS cases, no one is at fault. The unexpected death creates a feeling of waste, and the parents' deep emotional trauma and grief makes a SIDS case emotionally striking. Dr. Reznikov, who expressed a deep empathy for all parties involved in resuscitative efforts and who was himself the father of two children, became visibly angry when he recalled a resuscitative effort on a severely abused child: "This little kid was about eighteen months old. She was a beautiful child and someone just killed her.... That is hard to deal with. Every once in a while, I still think about her.... I still get angry with those people running around that can do that kind of thing to their child."

A second group of tragic resuscitative attempts are the efforts performed on patients whom staff members recognize. The resuscitative effort of a well-known sports coach or a prominent politician is often different because of the patient's highly visible position in the community at large. Thus, when Britain's Princess Diana died in a car accident, physicians tried external and internal cardiac massage for two hours, although her pulmonary vein—which carries half of the body's blood—was lacerated. As Dr. Thomas Amoroso, trauma chief in the emergency-medicine department at Boston's Beth Israel Deaconess Medical Center, reflected, "As with all human endeavors, there is emotion involved. You have a young, healthy, vibrant woman with obvious importance to the world at large. You're going to do everything you possibly can do to try and turn the matter around, but I rather suspect, in their hearts, even as her doctors were doing all their work, they knew it would not be successful." Other doctors agreed that "most other patients would have been declared dead at the scene or after arriving at the emergency department. But with a patient as famous as Diana, trauma specialists understandably want to try extraordinary measures."[18]

The tragic character of the resuscitative effort can, however, be more subtle. Information leaked during the resuscitative effort, for example, might gives the attempt a dramatic flavor. In the interview, a chaplain vividly remembered the guilt of a man with a amputated arm and hook hand who attempted resuscitative efforts on his wife. Also, when friends or family members greet the body after the resuscitative efforts, they sometimes provide information that gives the failed resuscitative effort more of a dramatic connotation. An ED technician recalled how she was struck when a widow told her that her husband had never taken off his wedding band in thirty years. Nurse Sarah Keller recalls:

> Two that stand out in my mind was the lady who was petting her husband's cheek, it was their first wedding anniversary and she was letting him go, and another one was a lady after her husband had died, and he was out playing basketball and had a massive heart attack and died as a young man. She was holding his hand, and she was saying she didn't know how she could go home and go to bed that night without him there.

Dr. Martine Chau explains why these resuscitative efforts become more personal and difficult:

> Well, it is definitely much more difficult if you see the family. If you are dealing with a patient lying there, then you can really

easily distance yourself. If you see the family come in and talk about, "Well, this was my father," or "He was going to have his seventy-fifth birthday next week." That really gets you.

A different kind of a tragic resuscitative effort is one in which the health-care provider, usually the physician, is blamed for the outcome. In this case, it is not during the resuscitative effort that the patient becomes identifiable but afterwards, in confrontations with relatives or in the courthouse. Dr. Chau recalled:

> MC: I had a very sad situation not too long ago. I think it was in the fall of last year, that a 53-year-old man had brought his 15-year-old son down to the basketball game. This was his Christmas present to his son. And he arrested. So the son called the [hotel] desk, and they called the rescue squad. This man came in completely dead. That was one other resuscitative measure that I just went on and on and on and on, trying to get him out of V-fib. And I knew there was no hope. But he was so young, and it was just a sad situation. Finally, we said that it is time to have somebody call the family and the wife, and the wife and two daughters came the next morning. I have never seen such hostility from anyone than his wife.
>
> ST: Toward you?
>
> MC: Toward me, saying, "I want my husband back." And I felt very bad. I felt like a failure because I had tried. And I went out of my way to counsel the young boy. We talked to him. He was absolutely in shock. The girls were very nice. She had one son-in-law with her, and he was very nice. I felt so bad until at one point I said, "Why am I feeling so bad? I didn't cause this. I am not instrumental at all." And I really was. I didn't know how to deal with that hostility from his wife until I myself talked to the counselors here. She would have to deal with it. It was her problem and not mine. I did what I knew to do. If I had just watched him die and not done anything, then I should have felt guilty.

A rescuer may experience and remember a resuscitative effort as tragic because it provided an experience that crossed the boundaries of medical science. Several years after the event happened, Nurse Marie Rivers was still puzzled about a patient who predicted that he would be dying. When she took care of him, he said, "If you lay me down, I am going to die." They put him down, and immediately he died. Several respondents confided to me that they believed that some patients know when they are dying. A respiratory therapist explained that she often can tell whether the patient knows from looking in his or her eyes.

> I think your subconscious prepares you. I still can remember the look in the patient's eyes, I am sure she knew she wasn't coming out of this. She just had a very . . . it was a look I hadn't seen before; she knew she wasn't coming out of this. I think your body somewhere prepares you for this.

Dr. Jim Atkins told me about a patient who was successfully resuscitated and talked about her experience as a near-death experience. When I asked him about an outstanding resuscitative effort, he gave me the following story, which combines two sets of tragic subcategories: a familiar patient and a boundary experience.

> I was at the hospital, rounding on the patients on Sunday morning. I got called by one of the nurses to see one of the patients who wasn't doing too good. When I got down there, she had arrested and was in shock. We started CPR on her, and within a relatively quick period of time she regained a pulse and did well in the intensive-care unit. The reason she stands out for me was, first of all, because I knew her for a while—seeing her in the clinic. Second of all, she had a near-death experience that was really important to her—a situation where she saw a bright white light and was walking toward that light, very peaceful feeling. She heard the voice of her sister calling her from behind. She turned around and saw her sister. She had been estranged from her sister for about twenty years and hadn't talked to her at all. She thought that she needed to settle this issue with her sister before she died. Essentially, she went on and called her sister and had a wonderful relationship with her sister for several years before she died.

I did not ask specifically about near-death experiences, and only two respondents volunteered those stories.[19] Many, however, offered anecdotal evidence that hearing is the last sense lost before death. Nurse Mabel Hall explained that this belief affects her reviving attempts:

> I really think that people are there listening. I've had a couple of people react if you talk to them during the resuscitation. Like

you tell them "now breathe, try to take a breath." They try to breathe on their own. They say hearing is the last thing to go, and I think they are right. I really think they are there, and they are trying hard, but sometimes there is not enough there to allow them to come back heart-wise, it is usually the heart.

Another nurse told me about a patient who had survived the resuscitative effort and came back to thank her colleague. He asked her why she was yelling during the resuscitative effort "to hit him again." The nurse had used "hitting" to indicate that the patient needed to be defibrillated. Apparently, the patient had heard this word while he was unconscious. A technician told me that he sometimes talked to patients to encourage them: "When a patient is in arrest, I sometimes try to tell them it is not time to quit yet—and come back. Sometimes there is nothing you can do about it except talk to yourself."

Tragic resuscitative efforts also occur when the patient beats all odds. In this case, the drama is the lifesaving event itself. According to common textbook knowledge, a patient should have died without oxygen for more than fifteen minutes, but a patient might regain a pulse after all. Or the patient might be on a roller-coaster with an upbeat ending; the condition improves and deteriorates repeatedly, but in the end the patient survives. During one resuscitative effort, a physician told the team a "thanatomimesis"[20] story, in which he and others thought that a patient was dead but, when they put the sheet over the patient's body, the patient suddenly regained a heartbeat. The sheet moved up and down. The team resumed the resuscitative efforts and eventually transferred the patient to the intensive care unit, where the patient died the next day. According to the respondents, cases in which the patient beats all odds are truly exceptional.

The Non-Category

Most memorable resuscitative efforts qualify as successes, failures, or tragedies. A fourth category, however, is one respondents consciously or unconsciously leave out. These resuscitative efforts are rarely mentioned because they are similar, or because they are not considered valid resuscitative efforts.

Questions about an effort's validity arise when the resuscitation team has been alerted or even has begun reacting to the call when the effort is called off. These are typically patients officially declared dead before much has been done for them. Patients in this category are declared dead on arrival in the emergency room or after twenty seconds or less of effort. The attempt is so short that the event is remembered only administratively as a resuscitation. Also part of this group are the false-positives. These are efforts in which the resuscitation-team members suspect that a bystander started unwanted chest compressions and mouth-to-mouth ventilation. Instead of a cardiac arrest, the patient may have been experiencing a deep sleep, unconsciousness, or a seizure.

Other resuscitative efforts that fit into the "non-category" are those no one remembers because "they all blend together as one gray blur." Each of these resuscitative efforts seems the same as the previous one. Some respondents put pulseless non-breathers in this category. These patients have a very slim chance of being revived, and the course of the resuscitative effort almost always follows the same pattern. An example of my observations,

> I am deciding whether I want to go running or take a shower when the beeper goes off. I rush to the ED to find out that the patient is still about fifteen minutes out. I check with the nurse who took the radio call. The patient is on dialysis, diabetic, and asthmatic. The paramedics have been giving two epis and two atropines. The rhythm went from V-fib to asystole.
> The patient arrives (black woman). Dr. Cole asks the paramedics, "Any luck?" They say, "No." "How long is she like this?" "For at least twenty-five minutes." The doctor then answers, "I might just call it here."
> He looks quickly at the patient and then says, "I just call it." The respiratory therapists leave. When the oxygen bag is taken off, fluid comes out of the tube. The paramedics say, "This could be the atropine and the epi we put down the tube."
> A dialysis doctor comes down to the ED. Dr. Cole asks if this is one of his patients. The doctor looks at her and says that he doesn't recognize her. He asks for a name, but there is no name yet. When the name is retrieved from the family, the doctor looks again and says, "Now I recognize her. She used to always wear beautiful flowery dresses." He takes off the sheet and looks at the patient. "Sure. She was very bad. She had everything—bad vessels, heart disease."

Like the physician who replied to me when I asked him about survival rates, "Can I throw out the ones that enter dead?" team members automatically ignore efforts in this "non-category" when they talk about resuscitative attempts. These efforts have no salient features. They make no lasting impression.

Some respondents did not have anyone in this category. A nurse told me that she vividly remembered every resuscitative effort and was touched by each of them. Other respondents claimed exactly the opposite. They (initially) did not remember any resuscitative effort at all. When I asked them to tell me about an outstanding resuscitative effort, they invariably gave me the last one in which they were involved. When confronted with my question, Adam Dinkes, an ED technician, answered, "Of all the times I have been involved in resuscitations, I would have to really strain to think about adult resuscitations, to try to remember them. I think it is a defense mechanism on my part." For Dinkes, blurring the particularities of adult resuscitative efforts was a way to distance himself from the intervention in life and death. His response raised an important issue: what do all these categories mean for the health-care provider? How do the categories help workers cope with their often futile interference in the gray area between life and death?

PERSONAL PHILOSOPHY

Different salient features allow diverse interpretations of the same effort. A patient with a somewhat regular pulse might be a success for a nurse supervisor, but the respiratory therapists might remember the length of that same resuscitative effort as especially bad. For the physician in charge, this same effort might be just another in a series of patients who stabilize for a couple of hours, maybe a day or two, but for whom the effort is forgotten after the paperwork is filled out.

Not only is the diversity of interpretations important. Also significant is the health-care provider's classification of the effort. Rescuers identify outstanding factors and convey meaning to the resuscitative effort. The interpretive spectrum that develops teaches the health-care provider an important lesson. Eventually, most team members will become, in the words of one nurse, "pragmatic" about resuscitations. As Nurse Carolyn Lanker summarized, "there is a code and a code." She continued, "Look, Stefan, I have been in nursing for twenty-seven years and have seen a zillion of them, and for so many it just seems an effort in futility. I think we should learn to let old people die." Many of my respondents expressed similar views. Dr. Chau explained,

I think I have acquired a more philosophical attitude: if it is time, then it is time to go. And a lot of that has to do with the fact that I have seen so many people die. I know medicine is not that progressed that it can keep people completely alive. It has made lots of advancement, and you are able to cure so many diseases. But the ultimate thing is that we all die. So my perception of death has changed. My perception of death, about it being a fearful thing, has also changed. Because it is the finality. I mean we are all going to die. So you grow up, and you accept that more.

These health-care providers reflect a personal philosophy about life and death, one that involves more than experience with resuscitation. Like the emerging nuances across categories of effort, such a philosophy slowly grows through an amalgam of personal and collective experiences. Taking care of sick family members, unexpected deaths in the family, a father who survived a resuscitative effort, working in a trauma center or an expanded ED, gaining more colleagues on a shift—together with five to ten resuscitative efforts a month over many years—all become part of a world view, a kind of wisdom about life and death.

This personal philosophy puts each resuscitative event in perspective. It serves as a meta-category: we can do the best we can, have a smooth effort with all the drugs given on time, perfect compressions and ventilations, but…. The personal philosophy fills in the dots. It provides a pragmatic meaning for the routines and the contingencies, for the miracles and the tragedies. Nurse Ruth Berns expressed her sentiment beautifully:

My attitude is that everyone has a time or date when it is time for them to die and it seems no matter what happens, some people survive when they shouldn't; the odds were against and still they survived, my feeling was that it was just not time for them to die. And it didn't matter what we were going to do for them. They themselves had that inner knowing that they were going on and live. And then there are some people who are going to die no matter if you did everything perfectly. It is their time to die. I always try to make sure that everything flows freely, but I know that if they die, it was probably their time to die, and if they live, although you try to hope that you helped them to live, ultimately there is something else going on, the person's will to live or whatever that mystic sort of thing. Yes, the numbers say they should have died, but it wasn't time for them to die.

The central aspect of this philosophy is an acceptance of death, a profoundly felt knowledge that the boundaries between life and death are malleable only to a limited extent. The health-care providers who reach this point accept that death happens and that they can do very little about it. They are ready to let go. Technician Dinkes reflected,

> I guess if I think of people who are good in the ER, those are people that are comfortable with the idea that death occurs, that death hurts, and there is nothing wrong with going in and saying to the family, "We've done the best job we can. We weren't able to save this person. I know it hurts you, and it hurts me, too." And to sit there and cry with the family. There is nothing wrong with that. As medical personnel, we are spending how many years of our lives trying to save people, and to admit that sometimes it doesn't work is very, very difficult for people. And for us to break down and admit that we are human beings is even more difficult.

Such a personal philosophy puts the reviving effort in a broader context of resuscitation theory and the patient's life course. Nurse Cybil Halperin explained,

> You do the best you can with whatever techniques and equipment you have at that time, but if it doesn't work out, it probably wasn't going to work out no matter what. A lot of it has to do with time factors. If you are too late, there is nothing you can do. So the thing is to start as soon as you can and do as much as you can right up front. If the patient is not resuscitable, then the patient is not resuscitable. It is not that somebody failed or something. It is a process that has, like with a heart attack, that has been going on for years and decades. It is the end point. It is very difficult to reverse what has happened to a patient for over fifty years. I think our job is to do the best we can, and if there is any chance of helping the patient, to go ahead and help them, but if things don't work out, then they didn't work out.

Several respondents wove religion into their philosophy when they stated that "God" or "the Man upstairs" has ultimate control over the outcome of the reviving attempt. Other respondents told me that the final outcome is to a certain extent "predetermined."

This meta-category negates the contingencies of resuscitative efforts. It allows the health-care providers to keep some distance from their involvement with someone else's life or death. Almost none of my respondents believed that the health-care team had much personal control over the outcome of a resuscitative effort. Most echoed the physician who said, "For a lot of these people, their outcome is written in stone before I ever see them." Ruth Berns noted, "You can't make a silk purse out of a sow's ear." Other respondents observed, "You can't make chicken salad out of chicken shit," "Garbage in, garbage out," "You can't pace a roast beef," "We're beating a dead horse," "You can't get blood out of a turnip," or simply "Dead is dead."

This pragmatic philosophy does not mean that members of the resuscitation team give up on resuscitative efforts. Their pragmatic view instead provides a rationale for giving each patient the best possible chance. For example, the ED technician Josh Brittan made both the pragmatic acceptance of death and giving the patient the best chance possible aspects of his personal philosophy,

> CPR is just an attempt. It is not an attempt for God; CPR is an attempt by humans to elongate and maybe sustain someone for a while. There have been people who have lived lives to the fullest after CPR. As a human, I think we have no choice but to persevere and save lives. I think that is one of the things that will never change.

Few people actually live full lives after CPR, but persevering is a part of the resuscitation protocols and the education of the novice rescuer. Most experienced rescuers therefore react against it and stress instead the pragmatic side of their efforts.

COMFORT WITH SUDDEN DEATH

When resuscitative efforts become routine, a deceased or surviving patient is not necessarily the most salient feature for health-care workers. The extent to which the resuscitative effort went smoothly, team interactions, the wishes of friends, relatives, and the patients might become instead the characteristics that the experienced health-care provider attends to and remembers. Even in tragic resuscitations, where the organization and technical expertise are overshadowed by the recognition that a human being is dying, death is not necessarily devastating.[21] In some cases, rescuers perceive the patient's death as a "good death" because of the course of dying[22] or because continuing or restoring life would be "worse" than death.[23] For other health-care providers, patients who should not have died balance those whom they managed to save. Still other health-care providers take comfort in knowing that they provided the best care possible.[24]

In some cases and for some health-care providers, resuscitations remain an emergency, but again, not always because death is about to occur. Some exceptional efforts might become emergencies for the entire staff. In one case, a homeless man was found in a creek in early spring and was severely hypothermic. To resuscitate him, the staff needed to warm the body because the body needs to be a certain temperature before it can be declared dead. The staff had not done this in years and was obviously frazzled by the procedures and the technology involved. In other situations, sudden death becomes especially distressing. During one of my nights as a volunteer, the ED received two groups of teenagers who had been severely injured in a car accident. After much physical and emotionally exhausting lifesaving work on the teenagers (some of whom died in the ED), nobody seemed able to deal with another life–death situation. I also met one nurse who did not like working in the ED and who, in her own words, "freaked out" with resuscitations. For her, every resuscitative effort was an "emergency." It did not matter whether she worked on young or old patients or had a smooth or difficult effort. The reason she did not like resuscitative efforts was that she felt that not enough was and could be done for the patient. Resuscitative efforts drained her; she could not leave them behind. Death was scary. She was looking for a different assignment.

The extent to which these exceptions stand out in the ED confirms that sudden death is generally not a terrifying occurrence. Health-care providers learn to perform resuscitative efforts with appropriate emotional involvement. Because of the high interprofessional character, the technical focus of the CPR training, and the fast initial pace of resuscitating, familiarity comes only after several cases. Eventually, the health-care provider learns to distinguish between "a code and a code." Some end up successful; others are bad, tragic, or uneventful. The result of years of resuscitative efforts is a pragmatic personal philosophy that puts in perspective the efforts of the health-care provider, the powers of medical science, the effectiveness of resuscitations, religion, and ultimately the finality of life.

The pragmatic philosophy and the rescuer's categories help maintain "detached concern"[25] in situations that otherwise would arouse the deepest kind of anxiety and questioning about suffering and mortality. This detached concern implies a level of comfort with sudden death, not just a distancing from death. In the ED, as in the outside world, the best way to distance oneself from death is to avoid contact with dying patients. For example, Nurse Ruth Berns, whose baby had died from SIDS, could not cope with attempting to revive babies and ardently avoided those situations.

Importantly, the personal philosophies shed a different light on social rationing (as described in Chapter 5). In the eyes of health-care providers, resuscitative efforts place them between a rock and a hard place. Instead of being moral enforcers, health-care providers view themselves as buffers between the wide availability of often futile technology, combined with strict legal implications and the unwillingness of relatives and patients to face sudden death. In their minds, the health-care providers do not cause the problems; instead, they try to manage ethical questions about lifesaving and protocol demands while keeping patient trajectories on track. Health-care providers have accepted that death happens and that death is not the worst possible outcome. The problem resides with the legal system that obligates resuscitating even if the patient is irreversibly biologically dead. The problem resides also with families and friends who panic and dial 911, unaware that they set the entire system in motion. Finally, the problem resides with people who refuse to discuss their wishes with regard to sudden death. The consequence is that health-care providers feel that they need to make decisions that other are unwilling to face. Their personal philosophy guides them in their decision making.

Pragmatic knowledge about death and dying helps health-care providers professionally, but their personal philosophy also contains an important message for the rest of us. Life is contingent. Death might happen suddenly, and not much can be done to postpone it. This personal philosophy comes from several interrelated factors typical to the work culture of health-care providers. Could some of the same considerations extend outside the medical domain? Pragmatism emerges in a hospital culture where people die regularly and everyone sooner or later comes in contact with deceased people and their relatives. Although a wide margin for improvement exists, it is unlikely that everyone in American society can accumulate sufficient death-related experiences to face sudden death comfortably. And even if health-care providers are comfortable with the deaths of strangers, they are unlikely to be as comfortable with their own deaths or those of their loved ones.

Although familiarity with death and dying definitely helps one to become comfortable with it, the more important factor is that health-care providers are in a position to act upon what they consider a successful outcome while knowing the limits of their actions. Health-care providers have a greater level of control over the reviving situation than others might. What makes a bad resuscitative effort "bad" is exactly the rescuer's inability to control the contribution to the resuscitative effort because of outside pressures or a subordinate position in the resuscitation hierarchy. For the other resuscitative efforts, if young physicians believe that an aggressive resuscitative effort is warranted, they can act on that belief. If nurses conclude that the wishes and needs of the relatives are more important, they can take care of family members and friends and invite them to greet the body afterward. If chaplains believe that a patient had expressed a wish not to be resuscitated, they can be part of the decision-making process. Conflicts and disagreements among the team members do occur, but staff can raise concerns and objections while the resuscitative effort takes place. Or if they remain frustrated, as in the bad resuscitative effort that took five hours, they can take their grievances to a superior. Even if the complaint process does not immediately resolve the issue, team members can excuse themselves from working with certain physicians. If the resuscitative situation looks hopeless, emergency workers can take pride in executing a flawless, smooth reviving effort. And if the effort does not work out as they hoped, they all know why, because they were there, they saw it, they touched and felt the body. They predict when their efforts might work and know when they might not. Practice teaches rescuers to scale back their expectations and still walk away satisfied. Although the protocols suggest saving lives under all circumstances, staff members can reappropriate the technology according to their own purposes and values.

The important lesson for non-medical people is that to increase our comfort with death, we should find ways to retrieve control over what happens to us and our loved ones when they die a sudden death. Norbert Elias reminds us that "death is a problem of the living."[26] But the living—who care the most and for whom sudden death matters the most—lose control once their loved one is wheeled into an ambulance. In the next chapter, I will suggest ways that relatives and friends can regain control and decision-making authority in the face of sudden death.

7   Saving Life or Saving Death?

RESUSCITATION ETHIC

AFTER CELEBRATING CPR for two hundred fifty pages, the emergency system researcher and physician Mickey Eisenberg becomes less confident and convincing at the end of his book when he asks the fundamental question:

> Should we attempt to reverse sudden death? Ultimately the only answer must be personal. And it must be addressed before the event, since those in cardiac arrest cannot make their wishes known. Most of us, I believe, would want to be resuscitated from ventricular fibrillation (assuming a basically healthy heart), but would we decide to be defibrillated if there was an underlying terminal condition (such as Alzheimer's or advanced cancer)? The answer is less straightforward. The point is that I cannot know what you want. I cannot tell how you value a few extra days or months of life. I cannot tell how you judge quality of life. In the face of no information, my obligation is to call 911 and initiate CPR. I'm not sure I have an ethical obligation, though I know it is a societal expectation. Personally, I would do CPR for a friend or stranger simply because I would feel too guilty if I didn't. But how much better it would be if I did know what you wanted.[1]

Of course, Eisenberg and his colleagues have fostered the "societal expectation" that lives can be saved, a notion that has promoted guilt if one does not engage in CPR. The resuscitation pioneer and advocate Peter Safar addressed similar questions at the end of his book on the science of cardiopulmonary cerebral resuscitation: "Is this [resuscitating] worth the effort? Can it be justified—socially, morally, economically? Is it supportive of human evolution on this earth?" Safar vaguely answers his questions affirmatively by pointing out that "compassion, reason and decency constitute a higher ethic than chance."[2] Like most physicians and emergency researchers, Safar and Eisenberg have argued that we should not resuscitate terminally ill patients, but that, in cases of doubt, we have an ethical obligation to opt for a full resuscitative effort.

After investigating out-of-hospital resuscitative efforts for several years, I have often wondered what I would do if someone in front of me suddenly collapsed. Would I start CPR? Although such a question might fall beyond the realm of sociology, I would feel remiss if I did not try to give my answer in turn. Safar and Eisenberg's answers are uncomfortable and vague because they consider resuscitating only in terms of saving lives. Their goal is to save as many lives as possible, but they are aware that some people cannot be saved. Where do resuscitation advocates draw the line? Their call for universal CPR would lose credibility if they grant that resuscitative efforts are futile under certain circumstances. I do not share their belief that "some CPR is better than no CPR." I assume that the possibility that simple bystander CPR will reverse a sudden death is greatly limited. For me, the issue is how I—and the dying person's relatives and friends—would feel afterwards if I were to walk away or if I tried to revive someone in cardiac arrest. The determining factors are dignity and compassion both for the dying and for the grieving.

The principle that guides my decision making is that resuscitative efforts are medically and socially warranted only under special circumstances. The medical indication occurs when health-care providers have an excellent chance to save lives. Resuscitation makes social sense when the staff turns a "lifesaving" intervention into a compassionate passing. But most situations meet neither condition and do not warrant the intervention. Instead of saving lives, we should try to save the dying experience, taking advantage of the opportunities and questions CPR raises. My purpose is not to turn back the clock two hundred years and retrieve a world without CPR but to imagine, as Leigh Star reminds us, that "it might have been otherwise."[3] I would follow four guidelines in my split-second decision making:

First, I agree that following the wishes of the person in cardiac arrest is most important. Unfortunately, few people make their wishes known in advance or have them visible at the time of an arrest. Second, I would consider the prospects for the person's survival. If the circumstances of the cardiac arrest were such that a life had an extraordinarily good chance of being saved (for example, a young drowning victim only two minutes underwater in a pool next to the hospital), CPR would certainly be indicated. Considering the low survival rates, however, I believe this list of indications is short. In most circumstances, even if I started a reviving attempt, my assumption would be that I would have no effect and that the person would be unlikely to walk out of the hospital and more likely to live on with severe neurological deficits or in a vegetative state in an intensive-care unit.

Third, I would follow the preferences of any relatives and friends (perhaps including myself) who are present. If they did not want a reviving attempt, I would not start it. But if they explicitly requested resuscitation, I would acquiesce, knowing that, for some, starting a reviving effort provides closure for sudden death and facilitates grieving, especially when significant others know that first responders and paramedics have done what they have been trained to do. Such attempts are already the unofficial policy for SIDS. There, a resuscitative effort is a complicated procedure for verifying biological and social death. It is done for the benefit of relatives and friends. I would also consider it my obligation to advocate on the relatives' and friends' behalf. If they desire, they should have the opportunity to be present during the entire reviving attempt in the emergency department. Such an attempt is different from the "slow" code performed in hospital wards because the staff fail to ascertain the patient's preferences with regard to terminal care and so "resuscitate" to cover legalities. Slow codes are medically, socially, and ethically inappropriate.[4]

Fourth, if no relatives or friends are present, if I have no personal ties with the person dying, if I do not know the person's wishes, and if survival is not a near certainty, I would follow the advice I once heard a paramedic give a colleague: "If I were to collapse suddenly, close the door and check back in twenty-five minutes." In most situations, I would chose not to start CPR, and I would make this decision in good conscience. I would decline to subject a dead person to an invasive and traumatic intervention. In this, I concur with Dr. Hendrickson, who explained: "In a better world they [the patients being resuscitated] wouldn't be there [in the ED] because there is nothing natural or sanctimonious about being declared dead in a resuscitation. It is far more natural to be declared dead with your own family in your own home. We have now taken that patient out of their environment, away from their family, brought that family to a very strange place that is very unnatural, only to be served the news that their loved one has died."

MORE EFFECTIVE CPR

A personal resuscitation ethic is a first step toward improving resuscitative care, but its potential for profound change is limited because it requires each of us voluntarily to make a difference. A more comprehensive approach addresses the problems that CPR builds into the emergency system and the protocol's indiscriminate, universal use. The major problem is that in the current system most resuscitative efforts are medically unnecessary and socially unwanted. Controversies continue in laboratories over whether universal CPR has the most lifesaving potential, rests on sound physiological principles, or is backed up with conclusive clinical and experimental research. Some authors suggest that the research phase for resuscitation techniques should be reopened. In field situations, resuscitative efforts rarely save lives but instead frame many sudden deaths as failures. The medicalization of the dying process renders us dependent on what staff members in EDs consider lives worth saving. Their well-intentioned attempts sometimes cause brain damage, and to avoid this outcome, health-care providers perpetuate disturbingly negative stereotypes about disability and old age. In turn, rescuers—both lay and professional—feel trapped by outside pressures to make the decisions that no one else seems willing to make. To protect themselves, they continue futile and costly procedures, and they suffer from guilt when a patient who was supposed to have lived instead dies. When considering advance directives, decision making at the end of life is distorted by the unrealistic portrayal of CPR on TV, the deception perpetuated in CPR-training courses, and the statistical juggling by emergency researchers. Advance directives further lack impact as health-care providers routinely reinterpret these wishes on the basis of what they consider appropriate.

The preferences of the people who have the most extensive personal experience with CPR underscores its problematic character. For example, in 1975, when the CPR pioneer William Kouwenhoven was dying, a friend of the family asked his wife, "Did you ever discuss what should be done if he doesn't...." Mrs. Kouwenhoven replied, "Oh, don't worry. We talked about this often. Bill always said that he didn't discover these resuscitation procedures for people in his condition." In a recent study, researchers have presented emergency health-care providers with a common forty-eight–minute resuscitation scenario having a relatively good prognosis and a reasonable time course, and ten of the 105 respondents declined even to have CPR initiated. Nearly two-thirds of those interviewed wanted to stop the reviving effort after twenty minutes. And only three preferred to be resuscitated for the entire episode.[5] In a similar study of emergency physicians and emergency system directors, more than two-thirds of the respondents reported that they would not want a resuscitative effort initiated for themselves, their spouses, or their parents if paramedics found them after an unwitnessed cardiac arrest, or even ten minutes after a witnessed arrest.

If the people who invented CPR and those who use it daily have serious reservations about its application—and if it generally fails to save lives—why don't we attempt to use CPR more efficiently? Cardiac arrests do not just happen randomly but are caused by years of underlying cardiac disease, often fueled by a mixture of lifestyle, environmental influences, and biomedical factors. As countless studies with low survival rates have shown, simply pressing on someone's chest, blowing exhaled air in the victim's mouth, or even jolting the body with electricity is not going to erase a long disease process. From a public-health perspective, it makes more sense to invest the resources of the current emergency system in programs to prevent heart disease and facilitate health care for all.[6] Many hearts are not "too good to die," but "too sick to live."[7] A life suddenly ended can still have been filled with unfinished but satisfying personal accomplishments and relationships. A sudden death is not necessarily a premature death; for some, it can be a timely death that avoided a lengthy debilitating illness. How can we make the emergency medical system more effective?

Eisenberg has proposed making resuscitative care much easier by determining in advance whether we want a resuscitative effort. My proposal takes Eisenberg's a step further. I propose reversing the current policy of initiating a resuscitative effort under all circumstances except when the person has a living will. Instead of a universal resuscitation standard followed in all but exceptional cases, resuscitation would become a special procedure performed for those who wish a lifesaving attempt. Instead of a living will, people preferring advanced resuscitative care would need to sign a "resuscitation will." Adult ACLS[8] would then be initiated only when someone had explicitly expressed a desire to be fully resuscitated. Administratively, this information could be conveyed by checking a special category on a driver's license application or wearing a health-care wristband. I imagine a system where, before deciding officially for advanced resuscitative care in case of emergency, people would be informed about the possible implications of their choice. They would be encouraged to talk to a health-care professional, who would explain the slim chances of survival, and the variations with age and disease, the possibility of neurological damage, and the medium- and long-term effects of resuscitative care. People would have choices about the kinds of life support they wish to implement in different kinds of life-threatening crises.[9] They would be invited to inform their relatives and friends of their choices and include this information in a health-care file. If sudden death occurs, advanced resuscitative care would be instituted only if the person had agreed to it or if the case met a limited list of narrowly defined, well-researched criteria with which resuscitative care has proved to be effective. Reversing the default resuscitation policy would make emergency staff liable for indiscriminate use of ACLS on the grounds that these interventions can do more harm than good. Professionals attending sudden death should be trained to inform onlookers, relatives, and friends compassionately that nothing more medically can be done to revive their loved one.

The advantages of optional resuscitative care are numerous, but most important is that the responsibility for a full reviving attempt shifts from physicians and other staff to the people who might benefit from the intervention and who have to deal with the aftermath if the resuscitative effort does not work out. The potential recipients of resuscitative care would thus preempt some of the ethical decision making and hidden rationing in the ED. This policy would probably also propel more people to articulate their personal wishes and foster an awareness about the process that takes place at sudden death. Unnecessary resuscitative interventions would be likely to drop dramatically with a system of resuscitation wills. Research has shown that people are less likely to chose resuscitative care once they are informed about CPR's survival rates.[10] In addition, the effort of writing a will, the legal liability for emergency personnel, and the potential economic advantages of decreased resuscitative and intensive care would probably lead to fewer resuscitative interventions. If advanced resuscitative care became optional, emergency system advocates would have strong incentives to make sure that resuscitation wills were honored. They would be less likely to ignore them, as many now ignore living wills. Finally, the consequence of eliminating much inappropriate resuscitative care is likely to be higher survival rates.

To make advanced life support even more effective, standards should dictate that when certified health-care providers find an adult cardiac-arrest victim in a heart rhythm known to be non-viable (such as asystole), advanced cardiac care should not be initiated. There exists no justifiable reason to pump drugs, electricity, and oxygen into a biologically dead body. Some members of the emergency community have voiced support for stopping unnecessary resuscitative efforts in the field, but only when initiatives to terminate resuscitative care in the field are combined with resuscitation wills can medically unnecessary and socially unwanted resuscitative efforts be circumvented, and only then can we restore control to all of us for whom CPR is intended.

Sometimes, by chance, an unnecessary resuscitative effort is avoided and offers an opportunity to witness what might happen if sudden death just took its course. I experienced such an event. My mother died when she was 54. She had suffered a severe stroke fourteen months earlier, and although everyone was aware that another stroke was possible, her death was unexpected. She had been stabilized for more than a year, and my family expected her to live months—if not years—longer. If she had died during the day and my father or brothers had witnessed her collapse, they probably would have panicked and called an ambulance, even though my mother had told us that she wanted to be a no-code. My family's region in Belgium has a two-tiered ambulance system: an ambulance with paramedics and a faster intervention car with a nurse and physician are sent simultaneously in cases of cardiac arrest. The physicians in charge are residents from a teaching hospital; they have scant emergency experience, and according to their own admission and stories from nurses and paramedics,[11] they resuscitate aggressively. If an ambulance had come to my parents' house, the health-care professionals would have started a reviving attempt, loaded my mother into the ambulance, and driven twelve miles to the closest hospital. At 54, my mother would have been deemed too young to die, and her death would have been similar to those I described in this book. After an agonizing half-hour in a waiting room, my father would have learned that his wife had died. Her body would have been transferred to the hospital's mortuary, and there we would have been able to visit her once, maybe twice, before the funeral.

Fortunately, that is not what happened. A visiting nursing aide found my mother dead in the morning on the floor next to her bed. She must have awakened that morning and tried to get up, but fell instead with a new stroke. The nursing aide followed my father's directions for emergency situations: she called my mother's primary care physician and my father, who was already at work. The family physician came to the house, certified that my mother was dead, expressed his condolences, and told my father to call a funeral director. When the funeral director arrived, he gave my father a choice: he could take my mother's body to the funeral home and keep it there until the funeral, or he could treat it provisionally, leave it in the house, and pick her up the day before the funeral. My mother stayed at home, in her room, in her bed. She looked beautiful, someone at peace. During the next five days, my father brought visitors into the room. They sat, cried, whispered prayers; some touched the body. Others did not want to enter the room. All the time, my father stayed with her and talked to her. My brothers and I joined him. It was a very sad and intense time. Still, we felt united in my mother's presence.

Of course, we wanted my mother to go on living. But I am glad that she was not subjected to an unsuccessful resuscitation attempt. Because of her terminal illness, my mother was not a good candidate for a resuscitative effort. My mother's death spared us the false hope that her life could have been saved if the resuscitation attempt had worked out. Her death was always an unquestionable fact. There was nothing particularly special or magical about it, or about our grieving. Our emotions did not match Kübler-Ross's theories; we were not following a particular Flemish tradition. Our actions were not inspired by Luddism or a hatred for doctors. Instead, we had relied extensively on medical technology and professionals during her illness and rehabilitation. When her death came, we just tried to hold on and let go in as dignified a way as possible.

EMPOWERING RELATIVES AND FRIENDS

While we aim for a society in which CPR becomes an option and sudden death is part of life, improvements can be made to the current emergency system. Universal CPR has been with us for the past twenty-five years and will not soon disappear. Its use is fueled by the same ephemeral optimism that makes lotteries successful. The odds of winning the $195 million Powerball lottery in 1998 were estimated at one in 178 million, and newspapers reported that people were forty times more likely to die falling out of bed and 320 times more likely to perish in a plane crash. Still, hundreds of thousands of people lined up to buy lottery tickets. In the same way, the prize of surviving CPR is very small, random, and highly valued. When someone suddenly collapses, people cling to the chance that their loved one will survive, and in the public imagination, the one survivor is stronger testimony to CPR's effectiveness than are the ninety-nine who do not make it. The possibility that a simple medical technique might reverse the dying process—like a deus ex machina,[12] which restores order at the end of a Greek play—is too powerful a cultural image to relinquish.

Because of the mythical quality of CPR, many deaths will continue to be framed by unnecessary resuscitative attempts. If we let go of the idea that CPR is primarily about saving lives, however, we will find ways to improve the resuscitation ritual. CPR has potential beneficial side effects: the resuscitative procedures, for example, take some of the suddenness of sudden death away. They offer the relatives and friends an opportunity to talk to a social worker or chaplain, bring relatives and friends together after the reviving effort, and provide solace that everything medically possible was done. If CPR is here to stay, the way to dull its sharp edges is to turn the procedure into a community-centered event that might ease the transition from life to death, making the needs of relatives and friends a central concern. CPR might then be about facilitating sudden death in a dignified and compassionate manner. As Chapter 1 explained, a dignified and compassionate sudden death implies that the possibility of death is made explicit, treatment choices are reached with all parties involved, the dying person's wishes are honored, and relatives and friends are included in the last moments, if not as care-providers, then at least as witnesses.

Empowering relatives and friends begins with creating a greater understanding of the dynamics of the emergency medical system. People need more honest information about survival rates in CPR-training classes, where CPR is still taught as a miraculous technique to reverse any sudden death. With a disturbingly paternalistic attitude, the people who construct CPR-training kits seem to assume that the public would not want to resuscitate if the limitations of CPR were widely known. During the AIDS pandemic, CPR educators have adopted the principle that "some CPR is better than no CPR," whatever the circumstances of sudden death. This philosophy creates seriously distorted expectations. Invariably, whenever I give a talk about CPR and tell the listeners that CPR rarely saves lives, an audience member comes up to me after my talk and tells me a heart-wrenching story of trying to save a stranger, friend, or parent with CPR. The rescuer tells of having failed, wondering what went wrong. Like Mark Lanchester, the paramedic in Chapter 6 who blamed himself for his patient's death, they needed to hear that lives can be saved only under exceptional conditions. Knowing this makes coming to terms with traumatic experiences easier. TV producers are unlikely to create shows around the failure of CPR, but such a depiction definitely would be more accurate. The closest we come to such portrayals in the media occurs when a celebrity dies after a lengthy resuscitative effort.[13]

People also need to know the implications of dialing 911 and the limits of living wills in emergency care. Although there is some regional variation, with emergency directors allowing paramedics different levels of autonomy, in general the moment you dial 911 the resuscitative effort begins, and there is almost nothing you can do to stop it. The 911 operator will summon an ambulance, and the paramedics have standard orders to revive unless obvious signs of death are present. In most states, paramedics do not have the authority to interpret living wills, even if they are shown or posted at the scene. They will therefore always start aggressive resuscitative care and transport their patient to the ED, where a physician must continue the effort until the protocols are exhausted. The difficulty with this system is that physicians are the only professionals who can decide not to initiate resuscitative efforts but they are not part of the ambulance team. Recognizing this dynamic, a chaplain admitted, "We tell people who have a living will or have been given power of attorney and wish not to be kept alive, 'If you have a heart attack at home, don't call 911. Don't call the EMTs because they are automatically obligated to do everything they can.'" Similarly, a nurse observed, "Our system somehow doesn't allow for calling the coroner instead of an ambulance or a doctor instead of an ambulance."

Because hopeless and futile reviving efforts demoralize everyone involved, several emergency directors have experimented with ways to include the physician at the beginning of the attempt.[14] In one of the hospitals in my study, physicians were part of the team on medically equipped helicopters. Physician John Cole described a situation in which his presence influenced the resuscitative effort:

There is another scenario. I should tell you about that. It happened when I was on flight duty. The patient was an elderly woman from a nursing home who was in a terrible cardiac shock. The only hope of survival would be to bring her to the hospital; maybe she could get on with a balloon pump. We went out to pick up this lady, and I spoke to the family. I said, "I'd like you to stay here until you have heard word that we have landed." They wondered why. I told them, "There is a strong possibility that your mother is not going to survive." They asked, "Aren't you going to complete the transport?" I said, "If she fails the resuscitation in the aircraft, I'd like to bring her back here. If she dies in the aircraft less than halfway to [the city], why should you travel eighty-five miles all the way to our ED only to have me tell you there that she died?" In fact, that is what happened. Five minutes after we took off, we were unable to have her rhythm going, and we went right back to that hospital and brought her to her family.... They reacted very positively. They appreciated that someone had thought about them and explained that she would-n't have gotten any better care either by our doing CPR all the way to [the city], which we wouldn't have done.

In this situation, the physician felt satisfied about avoiding a spun-out, futile resuscitative effort. The patient would probably have been de-clared dead in the ED after a lengthy resuscitative effort following the protocols. This event did not happen because Dr. Cole was part of the emergency response team, and he had the jurisdiction to send the heli-copter back, to take the patient to her family.

Elsewhere, paramedics transfer the patient's EKG rhythm through a telemetric device to the ED, where a physician can decide whether to transport the patient. The advantage is that a lengthy resuscitative ef-fort is avoided, but this situation might create new problems. An ED technician who trained paramedics added the following warning to such developments:

One of the aspects they are talking about right now is the poten-tial for stopping resuscitations in the field, which medically makes all the sense in the world to me. I would have no prob-lem with that. What I do have a problem is that I see how poorly we deal with death in the ER, and now you are asking people with much less medical training to handle it in the mid-dle of the living room, where the body is still lying there and the family right there is trying to deal with it. I think that is a terri-ble position to put paramedics in. We either train these people more, or we have to have a social worker there or someone else to deal with the family.

Indeed, stopping a resuscitative effort in the field does not make the dying process more dignified if no one can provide emotional support to relatives and friends or if no one claims the body.[15] A physician in Belgium recalled that the lack of professional guidance created complications there, because an ambulance cannot legally be used to transport deceased people. Because physicians are part of the ambulance team in Belgium, they regularly declare patients dead in the street. In a widely publicized case, a conflict arose between police officers and ambulance personnel about responsibility for the now-dead body. To avoid these situations, the Belgian attorney general formulated a compromise in collaboration with spokespeople from emergency organizations. Although the patient might be medically dead, the physician is not allowed to declare the patient legally and administratively dead. Because the patient is not "officially" deceased, the body can still be transported to the hospital under the guise of a continued resuscitative effort—even if no one performs reviving actions. The physician decides what to do on the basis of the place of sudden death and the "social condition" of the case.[16]

A second set of initiatives addresses patient autonomy. I have noted that ED staff routinely reinterpret living wills according to what they consider appropriate, so that the document's impact on the resuscitation effort is severely limited. Living wills can still encourage people to think about what they want done if they are incapable of making decisions about their health care. Ideally, living wills also stimulate conversations with loved ones about the possibility of sudden death. But living wills alone are insufficient. I advocate combining living wills with an assigned health-care proxy armed with a durable power of attorney, a signed, dated, and witnessed document that allows the proxy to make health-care decisions for when someone can no longer personally do so. In a resuscitative effort, such a person could be at the patient's side, arguing on the patient's behalf. Such an advocate would be much more effective than a document specifying preferences.[17]

Disappointed with the inadequacy of living wills and other advance directives, some people have resorted to tattooing their chests with "Do Not Resuscitate" in the hope that this message will deter paramedics from initiating advanced cardiac care. For example, *Newsweek* magazine published the decision of a 71-year-old woman to commission such a tattoo because she remained skeptical that doctors would follow written guidelines.[18] Medical observers discussing this policy have added that, to increase the validity of such an embodied directive, the attending physicians should tattoo their names as well.[19] Do these medical comments reflect irony, sarcasm, or "sound medical practice"? I am not sure. Much clearer is people's overwhelming frustration in trying to assert their preferences against the sweeping force of resuscitative care.

A final set of initiatives to dignify sudden death specifically addresses resuscitative efforts in the ED. As Chapter 4 demonstrates, most reviving attempts outside the hospital are communal events, and a resuscitative effort becomes more personal and socially meaningful at the end, when the physician has declared the patient either dead or stabilized. If the patient has died, the relatives and friends are encouraged to greet the body and say farewell. Earlier, however, when the patient's loved ones are kept in the counseling room and the staff goes through the motions of reviving in a separate resuscitation room, sudden death lacks compassion. Recently, this separation of patient and significant others has faced scrutiny in several U.S. hospitals,[20] where health-care providers have attempted to change existing policies and routinely give family members the option of attending the resuscitation. These new policies are hotly contested in the medical world. Articles in medical and nursing journals suggesting the presence of family members during resuscitations are guaranteed to draw a variety of heated letters from opponents and advocates.[21]

Harry Kochan, a social worker who did not routinely bring relatives into the resuscitation effort, recalled a daughter who had been unable to see her mother's resuscitation and returned a month later to complain in the business office:

> HK: She [the daughter] did not get in. Basically it was because of the timeliness of the person's death. They pronounced her dead within five to ten minutes of being here. She did get her mother registered, and I met her at the desk. She didn't want to finish registering: she wanted to go now to see what was happening. I told her, "You can go in. I assure you that you can go in. But we need this information first." We didn't even know who this woman was. Plus the staff, there were like fifteen people in there. There were just too many people in there. She couldn't have gotten into the room at that moment. Then the patient expired immediately. The physician came out and told her that her mother had died, so . . .
>
> ST: What happened then?

HK: She went in, and she stayed for about an hour. As a matter of fact, she is one of the family members who stayed the longest in all the time that I have been working.

ST: Then she returned a month later?

HK: It was because she couldn't get past that traumatic experience. She wanted to, and maybe she needed to go in.

To avoid situations like this one, certain health-care providers advocate that significant others should be allowed in not only after but also during the resuscitative effort. The prospect, however, poses potential problems. There were too many staff members in the room; the people at the front desk did not know who the daughter was; they first needed to register her mother; and the resuscitation ended very quickly. Weighed against institutional and organizational routines and practices,[22] the family's needs become secondary, but that need not be inevitable.

Family Attendance

The case for family attendance is usually made through the personal "crusade" of a chaplain, a nurse, or a physician.[23] The pioneer example is the staff of Foote Hospital in Jackson, Michigan. For more than a decade, staff members have given family members the option to attend resuscitative efforts. Reflecting on the way this policy started, Staff Nurse Cheryl Hanson and Head Nurse Donna Strawser wrote,

> In 1982 the staff members in the emergency department were forced to question the policy of excluding family members during CPR efforts by two separate incidents in which family members *demanded* to be present. One person, after riding in the ambulance during resuscitation, refused to leave the patient. Another begged to enter, even if only for a few minutes, to be with her husband—a police officer who had been shot. A chaplain stayed with the family members who were allowed in, and the first step toward changing a widely practiced custom was made.[24]

According to the Reverend Hank Post,[25] these situations were evaluated, and the staff expressed objections. Staff members worried about family members fainting, about getting sued, about the trauma of witnessing a reviving attempt for a loved one, and about the difficulty of resuscitating while a family member is weeping in the room. "This was a new and unsettling experience for the staff. They didn't seem eager to have other families witness their resuscitation efforts,"[26] Post explained. But a week later, the chaplain overheard a doctor remarking that if his wife were dying, "a herd of elephants" would not keep him away. The chaplain seized the occasion and asked why the doctor's wife would be different. The doctor acknowledged that it should not make any difference and agreed to a change in policy. Together, staff members developed a policy in which a chaplain or nurse would give family members the option to attend the resuscitative effort, and if they chose to do this, the chaplain or a nurse would stay with the family throughout the experience. This widely published experiment[27] has inspired other ED staff to try this policy in their hospitals.

Here, the needs of significant others receive the priority of, in the words of Dr. John Cole, "a second resuscitation" for the entire staff. Significant others remain informed of what is happening with their loved one during the resuscitative effort, and if they wish to, friends and relatives can attend the resuscitative effort. Skeptical care providers have participated in the new policy and report that it has changed their views.[28] Dr. Doyle of Foote Hospital described such a change,[29] "I was one of the more reluctant physicians. You have a feeling of being on stage.... As I see more family members, I think it's good for them."

How does this policy work? One chaplain of another hospital described the process at length:

> Usually how it works out is that family members arrive at the scene, at the emergency department, after the patient gets here. Resuscitation has gone on for some time, there is a certain rhythm. The initial confusion or initial scrambling around is done, and people are around the bedside—physicians and nurses. And because of that certain pattern, the flow, and because the family members are really pressing the issue of "I really want to see him, I *really* want to see him . . ., I promise I won't get upset, I really want to see him . . .," that is usually how the situation happens. Either myself or one of my chaplains or a physician and a social worker will go back and say, "Mrs. Jones, we are going to allow you to see your husband, and if you want to take your son with you. . . ." You can only take them two at a time, only two for just a brief instant. We try to tell you what you will see; we try and describe the room; we describe if he is intubated, and you'll notice if he is intubated we have what we call an advanced life support, what we call the

"thumper" moving his chest up and down, and we do that because his heart is not working, so we are having to do that. We are having to keep his heart going for him. We are doing everything we can, and he is alive, but he is alive because of our resuscitative efforts, and after a while, we will have to evaluate how much longer we can do this. But we will allow you to go in, you can touch him. We would encourage you to say something to him. And so that is how we set it up. And then the family comes in, and then it is very interesting to watch. It is like a parting of the waters. Staff backs up; it is like they open up, like doors opening up, so the family can get by the bedside. We normally get them near the head of the patient so they can touch and talk to the patient. And while they are there talking with their loved one, the physician will describe what is happening—about his injuries.

This experience differs from the policy at Foote Hospital in that relatives and friends there are explicitly asked whether they want to attend the resuscitation, and after ten years, the people in the community expect to attend the resuscitative attempt. According to a survey between 50 percent and 75 percent of the resuscitations are attended by family members or friends. Apparently, staff are most willing to allow parents to attend the resuscitation of their children and to allow relatives to appear at the resuscitative efforts of very old people for whom death was more or less expected. In all hospitals, a chaplain, social worker, or nurse remains with those attending, and if things escalate, the relatives and friends are asked to leave the room.

The presence of significant others during resuscitative efforts facilitates a difficult aspect of resuscitation work. The physician, who usually informs the family of the outcome at the end of an effort, has an opportunity to "break the ice" and communicate that news more gradually. The physician can build a rapport with family members. I found that staff members experience involvement with the family as one of the most challenging and rewarding aspects of their jobs. They therefore welcomed more responsibility. Nurse Jennifer Cohen explained,

I find dealing with families in times of death very rewarding. It is heart-rending, yet that is part of what I feel like what our purpose is all about. You feel like maybe we are trained a little bit more in that area sometimes than people in other areas.

The social worker Lauren Kaplan summed up why she liked helping relatives during reviving attempts:

> Knowing that I was there . . . providing emotional support and being there at a time in their lives when it was very critical and important to them. It is a moment that they will never forget. None of them. Some of it they won't remember; the details of it will go fuzzy as time goes by. But knowing that I have assisted them in making informed decisions . . . the rewarding part of it for me too is that they have to make decisions. Helping them move from "your loved one just died" to the point where they leave this environment and helping them feel that they were in control of something that happened here. They may not have been able to control keeping that person alive, but they controlled something that happened during this process, and they have some control when they walk out the door over what is going to happen tomorrow.

But this rewarding experience can also be very draining. Lauren Kaplan also articulated the difficulty of seeing a family grieve: "What is hard is it causes the medical staff to get in touch with their own grief and their own mortality. Many of our physicians don't mind that; it reminds them of who they are, but that can be uncomfortable for some." Therefore, at Foote Hospital, the chaplain checks back with staff members after a resuscitation episode, and, according to Hanson and Strawser,[30] "informal support networks among nurses have developed to allow them to talk about these feelings."

According to health-care providers, the most important benefit for relatives and friends is that attending the resuscitative effort allows them to come to grips with impending death. Dr. David Reznikov explained,

> And then sometimes I will actually take the family down with me and let them see what I am doing, because I think that what happens to most people is that one minute they see the family member, they are fine; the next minute, they are dead. . . . If you are fighting in war and your friend is next to you and your friend gets shot and dies, well, you have seen him die. So it is not just some vague concept or hazy notion out there; it is reality. And I think that the same is true with situations like this. I

think that if you see people doing . . . that they are trying to save people, you realize that they died. I think it is a step toward accepting it, and I think that is a big step toward getting over it. It is a problem a lot of people have.

Many health-care providers stressed that they had the impression that witnessing intense resuscitation work helped relatives and friends understand that everything possible had indeed been done. Several respondents recalled how relatives of patients felt guilty because they thought they should have done more. Being present, talking to the patient, touching while he or she might still hear or feel was regarded as very helpful. A follow-up bereavement program at St. Luke's Medical Center in Milwaukee, Wisconsin, shows that for family members the experience was "uniformly positive."[31] A similar follow-up program at Foote Hospital indicated that thirty-six out of forty-seven respondents, or 76 percent, "felt that their adjustment to the death was made easier by their presence in [the] room."[32] Thirty respondents (64%) believed that their presence was beneficial to the dying family member, and forty-four (or 94%) thought that they would participate again.[33] The same feedback also helped convince staff members in the hospitals where I conducted research. Liza Dolnik, a pediatric nurse, noted:

Some of the staff have a real hard time with it. It has taken a lot of talking as a group to be able to understand, and bringing back feedback from those parents that were there, about how valuable that was . . . for the staff to start to believe that this is a good thing. We have a real active bereavement program, and that does a lot of follow-up with families. We got the message very clearly from those families, that it was very important in their acceptance of the death. They were there, and they saw that everything was being done for their child.

Health-care providers did not anticipate the difficulties of allowing relatives and friends in the resuscitation room. They expected interruptions in the resuscitative effort, but the main difficulty happened on an emotional level: grieving with a family. The Reverend Dublin provided his perspective: "My experiences have been very, very positive. I have never seen a family member or family unit ever act out, get inappropriate with physicians, get angry. They will be upset and grieve, but never toward anybody, other than because of what is happening."

Again, this experience is echoed by the experiments at Foote Hospital: "In our nine years of experience, not one instance of actual interference with resuscitation activities has occurred. In a few instances family members were overcome with grief and felt faint or hysterical. The chaplain or other support person was able to escort them quietly from the room until they could compose themselves."[34] According to Dr. Doyle from Foote Hospital, the parents of one 16-year-old girl wanted to prolong the resuscitative effort. A consultant was summoned, and when he confirmed that nothing more could be done, the parents' objections ended. The risk-management specialist Judith Renzi Brown[35] argues that the fear of litigation is ungrounded because the policy allows strengthening the bonds between a staff and families and alleviates many doubts that could prompt a lawsuit. As a consequence, the General Assembly of the Emergency Nursing Association has approved a resolution in 1993 endorsing family presence during invasive procedures, including resuscitation.[36]

Most reservations come from a protective stance: resuscitations are too violent and traumatic to have significant others attend them. Significant others, however, have already been made partners in the resuscitation project outside the ED. Laypeople, especially family members of patients with heart conditions, are strongly encouraged to take a first-aid CPR course. Bystander CPR is the first link in the chain of survival of the American Heart Association.[37] In certain emergency medical systems, paramedics will arrive in the living room, on the street corner, or in another place where the resuscitation occurs and perform ACLS. These invasive procedures mirror the interventions of the ED. In many cases family members, neighbors, and others will be present, and sometimes they are asked to assist—for example, with holding a bag with fluids. In addition to these real-life experiences, popular American television shows regularly portray resuscitative efforts in detail. We might therefore question whether this protective stance is necessary or whether the current practice of separating the patient and family limits the family's choices for care.[38] One nurse supervisor wondered who benefits from the current practice of keeping family members in the counseling room during resuscitative efforts: "Sometimes I think that it is more for our comfort than for the comfort of the patients."

Family attendance situates the patient in a social network. It transforms an anonymous body into an identifiable person. The presence of relatives and friends who care deeply about the outcome restores humanity, compassion, and dignity to the dying process. With significant others present, the staff cannot readily fall back on disturbing distancing techniques—joking or merely going through the motions. They, too, must be emotionally present. Presence during resuscitation provides relatives with a sense of control. Resuscitating is about doing something in the face of death, and relatives can do something when they whisper farewells or encouragement to their loved ones, hold the body, stroke the head, or contribute to the decision to continue or stop. In most cases, the resuscitative effort offers them precious time to prepare and realize the inevitable. In these situations, sudden death has become dignified, not in spite of, but because of, resuscitative attempts.

Family attendance during reviving attempts originated within the medical professions. This reliance on health-care providers remains a point of contention. Resuscitation staff still decide when it is appropriate for relatives and friends to attend and when they should leave. Family attendance is thus most likely to work if the relatives and friends share the same racial and socioeconomic background as the staff. If ethnic differences are too great, the staff might redefine some displays of grief as inappropriate.[39] History also suggests another danger: a change in policy might be only cosmetic. Just as attendance of fathers during birth, the emergence of birthing suites, and the creation of birth-training programs has not truly demedicalized the birthing experience and the hospice movement has not profoundly challenged dying in hospitals, attendance of family members can become a mere consumer-oriented public-relations ploy if it is the only way in which resuscitative care is confronted. These efforts toward change lost much of their radical edge once alternative policies were integrated with established medicine.[40]

Another potential problem is that family attendance might become a normative expectation in which the staff redefines relatives who refuse to attend the reviving attempt as "bad" grievers. Such an overreaction would be comparable to the uncritical acceptance of psychological bonding at birth. Exhausted mothers who do not have the energy or simply do not want to bond with their babies right after birth have been labeled "bad" moms by hospital staff whom developmental psychologists have sensitized to the importance of bonding.[41] To avoid a similar labeling process, policymakers must make family attendance an option, not an obligation.

Asking for more compassionate sudden death from medical professionals implies that they will set the limits of dignified dying. Medicine's definitions of a "good" death will largely prevail. Fortunately, many ED practitioners seem to have accepted that death is inevitable and that they are not benefitting patients, their relatives, or themselves with drawn-out, futile reviving attempts. They realize, in Nurse Ruth Berns's words, that "nine times out of ten a resuscitative effort is more for the family's benefit than for the patient," and they are already looking for ways to avoid unnecessary resuscitation.

FINAL REFLECTIONS

Two centuries of resuscitation technology have changed the way Americans think about life and death; in turn, Americans have given new meaning to resuscitation. From an absolute end point of life, sudden death has become a malleable boundary guarded by emergency professionals. The result is a gap between expectation and reality: although every sudden death signifies a call for CPR, a generation of universal CPR has seen lifesaving only rarely. To bridge this gap between expectation and reality, we can try to chase elusive higher survival rates by turning every street corner, home, and beach into a twenty-four–hour satellite emergency department with CPR, defibrillators, oxygen tanks, and plungers to pump blood through arteries. Or we can create an infrastructure in which lives that have an excellent chance for survival can be saved while most cases allow a dignified and compassionate passing. History has shown that the first strategy has the appeal of a cherished but unattainable myth; most likely, it will remind future historians of Juan Ponce de Leon's quest for the fountain of youth or the alchemists' search for the elixir of life. The latter strategy, however, requires that we reserve CPR for true emergencies—when lightning strikes or people nearly drown—but do not rely upon resuscitation technology as a general defense against sudden death. Yes, some people who otherwise would have had a small chance of being pulled through might die. But resuscitation techniques come with promises only, not with guarantees about outcomes. If we do not have to save every life, we can focus on living life fully and letting go with dignity.

I have shown that, with all its problems and benefits, resuscitation technology reflects and furthers the meaning that different societies give to life and sudden death. The members of the Royal Humane Society made resuscitation possible while differentiating between apparent and true death and limiting their lifesaving efforts to drownings. With CPR

and ACLS, ED staff make resuscitation "work" when they balance protocols and legal requirements against pragmatic philosophies about the
finality of life. Resuscitation techniques keep evolving, and the opportunities for change and redirection are diverse. We must remember,
however, that we are all implicated in CPR and share the responsibility
to implement and support change for our own and our loved ones'
deaths. In the end, we always have the choice not to resuscitate and not
to be resuscitated, and we have the right to be present at the resuscitation attempts for others.

Appendix: Methodology

RESEARCH ON death and dying requires justification. The groundwork for this topic was laid when I was an undergraduate sociology student in Belgium. Inspired by the powerful book *Awareness of Dying*, by Anselm Strauss and Barney Glaser, I chose to write an undergraduate thesis on how nurses cope with caring for terminal patients. I approached this topic from an ethnomethodologically inspired theoretical framework and spent a summer as a student nurse on a pulmonary and a gynecological ward.[1] My research in Belgium became a defining moment. I enjoyed the ethnographic work and wrote about the complex negotiations around the hospitalized dying patient. My main finding was that, although nurses reported that they did not engage in terminal care, I observed them caring extensively for terminal patients.

The nurses I interviewed interpreted terminal care in the narrow psychodynamic way promoted by Kübler-Ross, and they failed to recognize the many other aspects of their work as terminal care. They took acceptance of dying as a normative expectation. While observing the lingering deaths of cancer patients in the Belgian hospital, I witnessed one resuscitative effort in which a physical therapist discovered a suddenly deteriorating terminal patient "who wasn't supposed to die yet." Resuscitative efforts were rare on the pulmonary ward, and the staff discussed this event at length in the days that followed. I was struck by Glaser and Strauss's observed difference between lingering and quick deaths and wrote in my field notes that it would be interesting to contrast the two ways of dying in contemporary hospitals.

I did not return to the sociology of death and dying until after I discovered the field of science and technology. During a summer workshop on interpretive theory organized by Paul Atkinson and Sarah Delamont, the post-doctoral researcher Tia Denora and my adviser, Jef Verhoeven, encouraged me to read sociology of science. Tia recommended *Science in Action*, by Bruno Latour.[2] Like many people of my generation, I found this book inspiring. It turned me on to the study of science and technology. I was fascinated by the theoretical challenges Latour offered when he blurred sociology's conventional understanding of agency.

During the workshop, Harry Collins gave an animated guest lecture on a weird spoon-bending experiment and paranormal science. Was this sociology of science? I chose a study of resuscitation technology as a compromise between the world of science and the world of medicine. Inspired by Latour, I was impelled to study how those techniques made the transition from the laboratory to the hospital.

Because it took me a while to figure out the best way to observe resuscitative attempts, I first started working on the history of resuscitation techniques. I reviewed the available research published in major medical journals; I also read archival materials at the Alan Mason Chesney Archives of the Johns Hopkins Medical Institutions, the Stanley A. Ferguson Archives of the University Hospital of Cleveland, and the Dittrick Museum of Medical History in Cleveland. I concentrated on the contributions of William Kouwenhoven and Claude Beck. In addition, I interviewed some of the key players in resuscitation, past and present, and read their biographical reflections. These primary historical sources form the basis of the first chapters, although most of my historical research has been published elsewhere.[3]

Before I could start my ethnographic work, I went through a protracted nine-month negotiation with a university and two hospital institutional review boards.[4] The boards in these two Midwestern hospitals were not used to ethnographic research. They raised concerns about studying "near-death" experiences and about possible liability. The most important consequence of this lengthy negotiation process was that I was not allowed to talk to patients who had survived CPR or to relatives of patients. This prohibition explains the focus of this book: I analyze how staff members make sense of resuscitation attempts. Over the years, however, I talked informally with several relatives about their experiences and have been able to glean more stories from bereavement studies. Still, my biggest regret at the end of this study is that I cannot match the experiences of the staff with those of relatives and patients.

In June 1992, I began my observations of resuscitative efforts in two EDs in a Midwestern town. The first ED was a level-one trauma center (the hospital had a trauma surgeon, neurosurgeon, and cardiac surgeon constantly on call), while the other ED was in a level-two trauma center (with less stringent staffing requirements and more limited services). Both settings were midsize community hospitals loosely affiliated with a university. One hospital also had a religious affiliation.

For an ethnographer, one of the problems with resuscitative efforts is their unpredictability. I had to find a way to be available without being constantly present. Rather than hanging around in the hospitals on certain days and waiting for cases to observe, I arranged to be paged whenever the staff was notified of a resuscitative attempt. Usually, paramedics would radio their arrival in advance to the emergency department. The departmental administrator would then page the non-emergency staff—the social worker, chaplain, and respiratory therapists. I asked to be paged, as well, and rented a beeper for my research. The administrator initially paged me separately, but later I received a beeper from one of the hospitals, which automatically included me in the paging system. Being included in this way enhanced my ability to observe, as I had already missed several codes because the department administrators did not remember to page me.

Because I lived about three blocks from the first hospital and five blocks from the second, I would ride my bicycle to the emergency department, and I usually arrived before the ambulance, so I was able to observe the entire ED resuscitative attempt. Because of the delicate nature of my topic (one physician compared resuscitating to sausage-making, noting that we all like sausages but would rather not know how they are prepared), I needed to establish a good relationship with the staff. I wanted to avoid the impression that I was evaluating individual health-care providers or that I came to the emergency departments only to extract data. I therefore volunteered in one of the emergency departments (the other did not have volunteers) and formed friendships with some of the staff members. In the first months, I also learned CPR and took an emergency medical technician course.

I observed 112 resuscitative efforts, approximately half the total cases, over a fourteen-month period (I missed resuscitative efforts because I was unavailable or because the staff did not page me). Of these 112 patients, 101 were declared dead at the end of the resuscitative attempt, and 11 were transferred to the intensive-care unit. I could not always follow the transferred patients, but I know that five died in intensive care, and I know of only one who was discharged from the hospital. Of the 112 resuscitative attempts I witnessed, forty-three patients were female and sixty-nine were male; ninety-seven were Caucasian, fourteen were African American, and one was Asian. My observations represent community hospitals, but they may differ from urban and teaching hospitals, which have a larger trauma-case load. My focus, however, was on non-trauma resuscitative efforts, typically for heart attacks and strokes, so the difference may not be that relevant.

After a year of attending resuscitative attempts, I felt that I had saturated the analytical potential of my observations and considered other sources of data. I had tried to take elaborate field notes during the resuscitative efforts, but after resuscitation was finished, the staff always dispersed, leaving me wondering what the effort had meant to the participants. I therefore decided to conduct a series of interviews with staff members. In total, I interviewed forty-five staff members. The sample consisted of nine physicians, fifteen nurses, three nurse supervisors, five respiratory therapists, seven emergency department technicians, two social workers, and four chaplains. Several of these respondents had worked previously or were still working as paramedics and offered reflections on that experience, as well. These care providers came from three hospitals—the two hospitals where I observed resuscitative efforts, and a larger urban Midwestern teaching hospital providing level-one trauma care.

In the first two hospitals, I selected respondents on the basis of my observations. In the other, I relied on a gatekeeper to select respondents. I tried to have the greatest variety of respondents: new and experienced health-care providers (varying from four months to thirty-one years of emergency department experience), positive and skeptical attitudes toward resuscitative efforts, varying ethnicity (two African Americans, two Asians, one Latino, and forty Caucasians), and gender (twenty-three women, twenty-two men). While I was writing Chapter 6, I became concerned with the fragmentary character of the interviews, and to develop a more complete picture with at least one respondent, I interviewed Ruth Berns, an emergency department nurse, on several occasions and elicited a longer story from her. Finally, for Chapter 7 I also interviewed a chaplain, nurse, and physician at Foote Hospital in Michigan but used these interviews only as background information.

The interviews consisted of fifteen open-ended, semi-structured questions using James Spradley's[5] technique of domain analysis. This technique applies three different types of questions—descriptive, structural, and contrast—to create a taxonomic framework for the topic under investigation. Descriptive and structural questions identified the full range of characteristics pertinent to lifesaving. Contrast questions generated distinctions between patterns generated by the other two types of questions. The interview guide covered questions about professional choice, memorable resuscitative efforts, definitions of "successful" attempts at reviving, family presence, teamwork, coping with death and dying, and ACLS protocols. The interviews lasted from forty minutes to two hours. As I promised the university's human-subjects committee and the review boards of the different hospitals, all interviews were audio recorded and later transcribed, after which I destroyed the tapes. To protect the anonymity of the respondents further, I have made all names of patients and staff in this book fictitious. In particular, cases in which respondents or resuscitative efforts might be easily identified, I changed the respondent's main identifiers or borrowed elements of several resuscitative efforts to construct one case. All this material was analyzed in the grounded theory tradition.[6] This data-analysis method is aimed at inductively building concepts that fit the empirical material based on a systematic comparison of coded interviews and conceptual memos.

While I was negotiating access to study CPR in hospitals, I unexpectedly received a phone call from my father. He told me that my cousin Ann had died in an asthma attack. Ann and I were one month apart in age, and as I was one month premature, we had long agreed that we should have been born on the same day. Although we lived in different cities and met only at family gatherings, we were close friends. We had often escaped the extended Christmas and confirmation dinners to talk about friends, parents, and dreams. Ann once wanted to become a social worker, but later became an high-school English teacher. Her asthma, however, was always a concern. Her room was furnished sparsely with synthetic material to keep dust out. She tried all kinds of therapies and saw an army of specialists, but nothing seemed to help. My father, who had been a severe asthma sufferer in his childhood, grew better in his late teens, but Ann's ailment kept interfering with her studies and undermining her self-esteem. Seven months before she died, she had been admitted to the emergency department with a severe asthma attack and had decided to try to master her illness through yoga and breathing exercises. It was during one such yoga session that Ann had her final attack. Her teacher initiated CPR, and Ann was rushed to the hospital. The staff worked on her for hours—to no avail. She died when we were twenty-four. I lost a very good friend.

Notes

INTRODUCTION

1. All names of emergency department staff and patients throughout this book are fictitious.
2. Cummins et al. (1991b: 1841). The emphasis is mine.
3. Because of the low survival rate, I will refer to resuscitative interventions as "resuscitative efforts" or "attempts" instead of "resuscitations." This book deals only with resuscitative efforts that began outside the hospital and were then transferred to an ED. The term used in the medical literature is "out-of-hospital" resuscitative efforts. I did not observe any in-hospital resuscitative efforts. I also disregard CPR for pets.
4. Anspach (1993)
5. Berg (1997), Bowker (1994), Clarke and Fujimura (1992), Epstein (1996), Haraway (1997), Latour (1987, 1993), Pickering (1995)
6. Huff (1954)
7. Myerhoff (1978: 213–14)

CHAPTER 1

1. Siebold (1992)
2. Kastenbaum (1998), Erhardt and Berlin (1974)
3. Stevens (1989)
4. Glaser and Strauss (1968: 203)
5. Freud (1918)
6. Kevles (1995)
7. Beeson quoted in Kaufman (1993: 259)
8. Gorer (1965)
9. Feifel (1959: xvii)
10. Ariès (1976)
11. Ariès (1977)
12. Ibid., 367.
13. See Berg (1997); Elias (1984); Starr (1982).
14. Foucault (1963); Illich (1976)
15. Not everyone agrees with Ariès' analysis. He has been criticized for his historical sources and conservative political message. See Elias (1984); Bourgeois and van Heerikhuizen (1980).
16. Fox (1981: 44)
17. See, for example, Corr (1993).
18. Fox (1979)

19. Glaser and Strauss (1965, 1967, 1968)

20. de Beauvoir (1965: 45)

21. Ibid., 101.

22. Sudnow (1967)

23. Mitford (1963)

24. Siebold (1992: 58)

25. Anonymous organizer in 1982, quoted in Paradis (1985: 6)

26. Rinaldi and Kearl (1990)

27. The most important are *Omega* and *Death Education,* later renamed *Death Studies.*

28. In 1964, Robert Fulton found only four hundred citations for a bibliography on the subject on death and dying; by 1977, he could list 3,800 titles. See Fulton (1977).

29. Lofland (1975: 10)

30. Siebold (1992)

31. This created a problem opposite to that of the past: instead of not being informed at all, patients were over-informed. "Truth dumping" became the new issue.

32. Stoddard (1978); Riesman (1935)

33. Already by 1890, Rose Hawthorne Lathrop (daughter of Nathaniel Hawthorne) had organized a group of women as "Servants of Relief of Incurable Cancer" in the United States. This group became later the Dominican Sisters of Hawthorne and worked out of six facilities: Siebold (1992).

34. Wald (1996)

35. Hospice care did not automatically become accepted in this country. See Siebold (1992) for the translation work that needed to be done between the health-care systems of the United Kingdom and the United States.

36. Hamilton and Reid (1990)

37. Neither do strokes or Alzheimer's disease fit into the hospice paradigm, because people in those conditions can easily live for several years. Kübler-Ross, who has been suffering from strokes, is not eligible for hospice care.

38. Dempsey (1975: 232–233)

39. Munley (1983: 52)

40. Mor (1987)

41. Siebold (1992: 137)

42. Quill (1993)

43. Miller (1992)

44. Humphry (1978). The "slippery slope" and abandonment of the dying who choose assisted suicide became apparent when Humphry's second wife, Ann Wickett, took her own life. She reported that Humphry had left her three weeks after her cancer surgery and divorced her. She left a suicide note for Humphry, stating in part, "Ever since I was diagnosed as having cancer, you have done everything conceivable to precipitate my death. I was not alone in recognizing what you were doing. What you did—desertion and abandonment and subsequent harassment of a dying woman—is so unspeakable there are no words to describe the horror of it." Gabriel (1991: 6).

45. Humphry(1991)

46. Kevorkian (1991)

47. Quill (1991)

48. Quill (1996)

49. In Oregon, the patient's request for assisted suicide must be in writing and witnessed by an Oregon resident 18 years old or older. A consulting physician must certify that the patient's condition is terminal, and a fifteen-day waiting period must occur between the patient's request and obtaining the suicide prescription. The physician must ensure that the patient's decision is voluntary by providing information about diagnosis, prognosis, and other options such as hospice or comfort care, and referral to a state-licensed psychologist or psychiatrist if depression is suspected. The request must first be made in conversation with the physician, then put in writing, witnessed by two people, one of whom is not a relative or heir of the patient. At the time that the medication is prescribed, the physician must again verify that the patient is making an informed decision.

50. Mairs (1996: 122)

51. In the mid-seventies, the Karen Ann Quinlan case had resulted in a slew of state initiatives. The Patient Self-Determination Act, in turn, grew out of a highly publicized legal case: the life and death of Nancy Cruzan, a young woman from Missouri who became comatose after a car accident in 1983. Three years after the accident, she did not show the slightest signs of improvement, and her parents asked to have the feeding tubes that kept her alive removed. Without Nancy's consent, physicians were uncomfortable ending treatment, and the state attorney's office was asked to rule on the case. A trial court ruled that Nancy Cruzan had a fundamental right to refuse or accept the withdrawal of "death-prolonging procedures." The Missouri attorney general appealed this ruling to his state's Supreme Court. By a 4–3 margin, the lower court's ruling was overturned. A key factor in this decision was that Nancy had not prepared a living will, although she had expressed her general intent in a conversation with a close friend a year previously. She had told the friend that if very ill, she would not want to continue her life unless she could live "at least halfway normally." The U.S. Supreme Court agreed to consider the parents' appeal of the Missouri Supreme Court decision. By a 5–4 margin, the nation's highest court refused to overturn the state's decision. Each state has the right to establish due process in order to safeguard the rights of all those involved. Nancy Cruzan had the right to refuse "death-prolongation" procedures, but the State of Missouri had the right to require what it considered to be clear and convincing evidence that this would really have been Cruzan's intentions if she could express herself. The Supreme Court created a way out of the problem. The state could reconsider the evidence and approve withdrawal of life-support activities. That is what happened when Nancy's physician changed his mind and agreed that it was not in the patient's interest to continue the tube feeding and hydration. Nancy Cruzan died quietly on December 26, 1990, twelve days after the tubes were removed.

52. Berger (1993)

53. Kastenbaum (1998)
54. Lattin (1997)
55. Anspach (1993: 166)
56. Moller (1990: 37)
57. Ibid., 32–34.
58. Illich (1976: 206)
59. Mannes (1973: 31)
60. Fletcher (1977: 355)
61. Cassell (1976: 459); Benoliel (1987: 174)
62. Thompson (1984: 227)
63. Campbell (1979: 330)
64. Illich (1976: 205)
65. Veatch (1991: 52)
66. Munley (1983: 5)
67. Kevorkian (1991)
68. Sontag (1978)
69. Kastenbaum (1993)
70. Callahan (1993: 195–96)
71. Kellehaer (1990)
72. Kastenbaum and Normand (1990: 216)
73. Bury (1997: 168)

Chapter 2

1. See Comroe (1979a); Cooper (1975); Eisenberg (1997).
2. Holy Bible, Authorized King James Version. II Kings (4: 32–37)
3. Fragmentary records also testify that different cultures tried widely diverse ways to mold the border between life and death. Ancient people realized that the loss of body heat is one attribute separating life from death. Therefore, warm ashes, burning excrement, hot-water bottles and blankets were placed directly on the victim. American Indians believed that smoke contained the spirits of life and attempted to revive the dead by insufflation of smoke into the rectum using an animal bladder. An alternative set of efforts included trying to wake the victim from a "deep sleep." Yelling, crying, loud noises, hitting, slapping, and whipping were tried. Early Russians buried their victims upright with the head and chest exposed and splashed water on the face. With the possible exception of midwives using mouth-to-mouth ventilation on newborns to clear their nostrils from mucus, none of these methods was practiced on a wide scale: Liss (1986).
4. Barry (1804: 18)
5. The society, De Maatschappij tot Redding van Drenkelingen Amsterdam, is still active.
6. What follows is based partly on the three Hunterian Lectures by Arthur Keith delivered March 1, March 3, and March 5, 1909, in the Theatre of the Royal College of Surgeons in England and published in *The Lancet* on March

13, 1909. Dr. Keith was, at that time, Hunterian Professor and Conservator of the Museum of the Royal College of Surgeons of England. For the three lectures, he reviewed the archival material of the Royal Humane Society. In addition, I also consulted some of the annual reports of the Royal Humane Society in the National Archives.

7. Hawes (1778: 23). Hawes's critical review of the way the "Mortality Bills" were collected in 1782 gives some insight into the prevalent causes of death and the theories of death. In that year, 1,193 people died, six hundred of whom died from old age. Three people died from grief, fifty-six were "Lunatick," four died from excessive drinking, two children were "overlaid" by their mothers, and 496 others, mostly children, died from "teeth" (they presumably died when their teeth started growing). Eleven people were executed that year, one person died from dog bites, and there were still 125 drownings (Hawes 1783).

8. Royal Humane Society (1809). Emphasis in original.

9. Shapin and Schaffer (1985)

10. Royal Humane Society (1803)

11. Fothergill (1795: 17)

12. Strive (1803: 658–62)

13. Barry (1804)

14. Shakespeare, *Pericles*, Act III, Scene II. The Royal Humane Society would quote the first sentence (until "overpressed spirits").

15. By 1809, the Royal Humane Society had chapters or sister societies in the following cities: Birmingham, Bristol, Exeter, Gloucester, Kingston upon Hull, Lancaster, Northampton, Milton Mowbray, Newcastle upon Tyne, Norwich, Shropshire, Whitehaven, Wisbeach, Bath, Leicester, Eastern Coast, York, Rivers Wreak and Eye, Folmouth, Suffolk, Bedford, Aberdeen, Glasgow, Leith, Mantrase Forth and Chyde Navigation, North Whales, Swansea, Dublin, Cork, Madras, Calcuta, Hallifax, Nova Scotia, Jamaica, Amsterdam, Berlin, Forlitz, Prague, Copenhagen, St. Petersburgh, Algiers, Pennsylvania, Boston, New York, and Baltimore (Royal Humane Society, 1809).

16. Yates (1807: 26–27)

17. Keith (1909: 897)

18. The Royal Humane Society is not only the precursor of resuscitation techniques but also the forerunner of first-aid organizations, particularly the Coast Guard. The society designed lifesaving boats, mortars to shoot rescue lines to foundering ships, and a variety of drags and hooks to retrieve people from the water or from under the ice.

19. Fumigation required that the rescuers blow tobacco smoke rectally into the victim. Arthur Keith wrote that "sometimes all passengers on a Dutch canal boat might be summoned to assist the operator in administering this means if the special instrument, the fumigator, was not available": Keith (1909: 898).

20. This method was recommended in one of the first first-aid books, *Helps for Suddain Accidents Endangering Life.* published in 1633 in London. The author, Dr. Stephen Bradwell, recommends: "Turn the feete upward, head and mouth downward and so hold by the heels that the water may come out. Let others help forth the water by stroaking, crushing, and driving his belly and stomach

reasonably hard, from the bottom of his belly toward his throat. If it be cold weather let all this be done in a warme roome before a good fire."

21. Keith (1909: 898)

22. Fothergill (1795)

23. Two people for artificial respiration, two for electrical operation, two for friction, one to haul stuff.

15 steps:

1. dry body
2. use bellows for artificial respiration
3. electrical machine
4. stimulate cordial in stomach
5. stimulate enemas
6. friction body, position bladder of tepid water
7. warm bath
8. take temperature
9. stimulate sensory organs (smell, hearing, sound)
10. continue intermittently with artificial respiration–electricity
11. moderate stimulating powers when life is restored
12. continue this for 3 hours
13. if no medical assistance, focus on respiration
14. put patient in bed
15. if fever, moderate bleeding

24. The machine was used in the following way: "[Put] one discharging rod just below the right breast, other above the short ribs of the left. Electrometer being moved a quarter of an inch from the jar, let the electrical current be passed directly through the heart. The electrical shock being given, let the lungs be emptied by making an expiration with the double bellows, or by suffering the air to escape by mouth, while gentle pressure is made on the chest": Fothergill (1795).

25. Hawes (1793)

26. Schechter (1969)

27. Vesalius (1543)

28. Dalrymple quoted in Keith (1909)

29. Keith (1909: 748)

30. Hall (1857)

31. Silvester (1858)

32. Keith (1909: 826)

33. Laborde (1894)

34. Keith (1909: 895)

35. Edward A. Schafer (or Sharpey-Schafer or Shäfer) (1850–1935) was elected fellow of the Royal Society when he was only 28 years old; he served as Jodrell professor at University College. then became a professor at Edinburgh University. He was a co-discoverer of epinephrine, but is equally well known for his physiological studies of the pituitary gland, the neurone, and the localization of cerebral functions. See Star (1989) and Clarke (1998) for Schafer's role in the latter research program.

36. Keith (1909: 828)

37. Schafer describes his instrument in the following passage: "The apparatus which was used in the experiments referred to in the report consisted of a counterpoised bell-jar filled with air and inverted over water; to or from this the air of respiration was conducted from the mouthpiece (or mask) by a curved tube which passed through the water and opened the bell-jar. When, therefore, air was drawn by the movement of inspiration from the bell-jar this sank in the water, and when air was forced into it by the movement of expiration it rose. These movements of the bell-jar were recorded upon a slowly moving blackened cylinder, and the diameter and corresponding cubic contents of the bell-jar being known, the amount of air exchange was found by measuring the ordinates of the curves described on the cylinder": Schafer (1903: 40).

38. Karpovich (1953: 57)

39. Schafer (1904)

40. I am puzzled with Comroe (1979b): how can a method increase its tidal volume if one takes measurements for five minutes instead of with each breath?

41. See Comroe (1979a, 1979b, 1979c)

42. Ross (1945)

43. Ibid.

44. The author cautions about the validity of the results. There is no information on the time lapse between asphyxia and the start of treatment; several methods were used simultaneously, and therefore not enough information exists to evaluate individual methods.

45. With hindsight, David Cooper suggested that the chant, "Out goes the bad air, in comes the good air," should have been, "Nothing is going out, and nothing is coming in": Cooper (1975: 491).

46. To compare the face-up and face-down position, Gordon and his collaborators had equipped eight of the fresh corpses with a mouthpiece and closed the nostrils with a clip. This provided an airtight airway and, at the same time, permitted the tongue and the mandible to remain free. In the back-pressure arm-lift and the back-pressure hip-lift methods, there were no blockages of the airway, whereas in the Silvester method, the airway was blocked in four of the eight cases.

47. Gordon et al. (1951)

48. Dill (1951)

49. Elam et al. (1958); Safar (1959)

50. I interviewed Dr. Safar, and (probably to test me) he asked me in the beginning of the interview what I considered his most important achievement in the field of resuscitative efforts. Peter Safar has an exceptionally distinguished research record in the field of resuscitation science. He has been involved in most of the research of the past decades; even now in retirement, he is still part of research projects on brain resuscitation. I told him that in my opinion it was the research on clearing the airway. He wholeheartedly agreed—and was slightly surprised that I knew this. The interview went very amicably after that.

51. Like most researchers in military institutions, Cooper complained about the security checks, lack of enthusiasm over one's work, short work hours, and reveille cannon: Cooper (1975: 493).

52. In his article, the report was dated in August 1957. However, from the context of his story, the report should have been written in August 1950: Johns and Cooper (1957).

53. Elam (1975: 263)

54. Johnny Elder and Elwyn Brown

55. Elam (1975: 265)

56. Ibid.

57. Elam et al. (1954)

58. Greene et al. (1956)

59. Gordon et al. (1958)

60. Dill (1958: 318)

61. In retrospect, it is striking that mouth-to-mouth ventilation did not make the list of methods in 1948 to be tested, even though isolated researchers continued to recommend it. In 1943, Ralph Waters published an article on simple methods for artificial respiration in the *Journal of the American Medical Association* and mentioned:"Direct inflation of the lungs is always at hand. Either the nose or the mouth may be blown into while one hand of the rescuer holds the other portal closed. The other hand, resting on the subject's chest, perceives the point at which the lungs are sufficiently inflated": Waters (1943). Also, Cecil Drinker (1945) wrote about mouth-to-mouth ventilation: "The most ancient method for restoring breathing is mouth-to-mouth insufflation—a method which, in my opinion, will always be one of the best." A member of the NAS-NRC resuscitation team, Motley, mentioned the need to consider mouth-to-mouth method. This suggestion was not carried further because the objection was raised that expired air was too low in O_2 and too high in CO_2. A second objection was that breathing against the airway resistance and elastic recoil of the victim's lungs and thorax would exhaust the rescuer. Third, the researchers feared that a large rescuer could overinflate the lungs of a small victim. Reflecting back, Comroe speculated that without a cure for tuberculosis, the real reason why the researchers did not test the method was the fear of infection transmitted by a dying stranger. Comroe (1979b: 1028).

62. Gordon (1967: 23). However, Safar (1975b) mentions that the findings for adults were only preliminary in the first conference and that only at a second conference were all the findings of the research available.

63. Again, this is ironic because mouth-to-mouth ventilation started in the field of midwifery.

64. The last part of this chapter is based on interviews and archival research in the Alan Mason Chesney Medical Archives of the Johns Hopkins Medical Institutions. The discovery was actually more a rediscovery. The technique had been described previously at several points in the literature but had never caught on.

65. Early observers compare the visual effect to a bag of wriggling worms.

66. Kouwenhoven Papers, Alan Mason Chesney Medical Archives of the Johns Hopkins Medical Institutions, box 905, no. 478.

67. Kouwenhoven, Jude, and Knickerbocker (1960: 1066)

68. Ibid., 1064.

69. Kouwenhoven (1966: 272). Italics in original.

70. This is more extensively discussed in my dissertation: Timmermans (1995a).

71. See Beck and Kouwenhoven correspondence, Alan Mason Chesney Archives of the Johns Hopkins Medical Institutions.

72. Benson (1961)

73. Jude, Kouwenhoven, and Knickerbocker (1964: 59)

74. See Collins (1983)

Chapter 3

1. Winchell and Safar (1966)

2. Jude, Kouwenhoven, and Knickerbocker (1961a; 1961b); Morgan (1961); Klassen et al. (1963); Demos and Poticha (1963); Baringer et al. (1961); and Clark (1962)

3. Jude, Kouwenhoven, and Knickerbocker (1964)

4. Editorial (1962)

5. Jude, Scherlis, and Farr (1961)

6. Clark (1962: 338)

7. Lind and Stovner (1963: 933)

8. NRC-NAC (1966: 197)

9. Rogers (1966)

10. Leighninger (1975). Ironically, several medical organizations are now strong promoters of similar voluntary organizations. The American Heart Association, for example, organizes the Citizen CPR Foundation, Inc.

11. Editorial (1965)

12. The list went even further. According to a 1965 Red Cross poster, "E" referred to "EKG"; "F" to "fibrillation treatment"; "G" to "gauge"; "H" to "hypothermia"; and "I" to "intensive care."

At the last CPR-ECC conference, the "ABC" idea was revisited, but this time "ABCD" (together with the chain-of-survival idea and the ten commandments of CPR) became the gimmick of the revision. The "D" stands for "defibrillation": American Heart Association (1994).

13. NRC-NAC (1966: 195)

14. Kouwenhoven to M.F. Brown, October 12, 1964. Kouwenhoven Papers. Alan Mason Chesney Archives of the Johns Hopkins Medical Institutions, box 912.

15. Haller (1990)

16. Sudnow (1967: 100)

17. Pantridge and Geddes (1967: 272)

18. Nagel et al. (1970: 336)

19. Grace and Chadbourn (1969)

20. Crawley, Lewis, and Ailshie (1975)

21. CPR-ECC (1973)

22. Killip (1968). Social scientists have questioned the advantages of costly coronary-care units: see Waitzkin (1979).

23. See Jude, Kouwenhoven, and Knickerbocker (1964), or Adgey et al. (1969)

24. Adgey et al. (1969)

25. CPR-ECC (1973: 864)

26. Ibid.

27. Beck and Leighninger (1959; 1962)

28. Other countries such as Belgium have a resuscitation registry: Martens and Vanhaute (1994). In the United States, Stephenson set up a registry for open-heart cardiac massage in the fifties: see Stephenson (1974).

29. Eisenberg et al. (1990a)

30. Ibid., 185.

31. Eisenberg et al (1990b: 1250)

32. Cummins et al. (1991a)

33. Cummins (1993: 38)

34. Hedges (1993)

35. Becker (1993: 2)

36. Cummins et al. (1991a: 963)

37. See, for example, Becker et al. (1993: 601); Gallagher et al. (1995: 1923); Swor et al. (1995).

38. Gallagher et al. (1995: 1923)

39. Gallagher et al. (1995)

40. Swor et al. (1995)

41. Sweeney et al. (1998)

42. Becker et al. (1993). I will discuss the race, sex, and socioeconomic-status differences of CPR survival in Chapter 5.

43. Niemann (1993: 8)

44. Cummins et al. (1991b)

45. In the resuscitation literature, the Seattle and King County, Washington, survival rate tends to increase to mythical proportions. Some researchers quote a survival rate ranging anywhere from 30 percent to 40 percent for Seattle: see, for example, Haynes et al. (1991).

46. Eisenberg (1992: 1123)

47. The only other place that seems to have been able to replicate and even outdo Seattle's results is San Juan Island: Killien et al. (1996). The survival rate on this rural island of 5,000 inhabitants—where no one is ever farther than six miles from the hospital—for witnessed cases of ventricular fibrillation and ventricular tachycardia was 43 percent. Interestingly, only one out of twenty-eight persons survived when the cardiac arrest took place beyond a two-mile range around the hospital. Sixteen out of forty-seven people who had suffered cardiac arrest within the two-mile range were discharged alive.

48. Becker et al. (1993: 605). The emphasis is mine.

49. Lombardi, Gallagher, and Gennis (1994)

50. Weaver (1991)

51. Gray, Capone, and Most (1991)

52. Ibid., 1397.

53. Cummins et al. (1991b)

54. Eisenberg et al. (1980)

55. Haynes et al. (1991)
56. Olson et al. (1989)
57. See Kellerman et al. (1993); Sweeney et al. (1998)
58. Sweeney et al. (1998: 240)
59. Pepe, Abramson, and Brown (1994: 1037)
60. Ginsburg (1998)
61. Cummins (1995: 836)
62. Cummins's call is not well heeded by his colleagues: Swor et al. (1995) and Gallagher et al. (1995) still wonder whether bystander CPR indeed makes a difference for survival.
63. Bossaert et al. (1989)
64. Asystole and electromechanical dissociation (EMD) are heart rhythms.
65. Swor et al. (1995)
66. Gray, Capone, and Most (1991)
67. Miranda (1994: 524)
68. Berek et al. (1995: 544–45)
69. Ronco et al. (1995)
70. I am assuming that most patients did not have neurological deficits before they were resuscitated. Information about the neurological state before the resuscitative intervention was not available.
71. Graves et al. (1997)
72. Safar (1993: 325)
73. Tisherman et al. (1997)
74. Tang et al. (1997); Safar (1975a)
75. Weil and Tang (1997: 449)
76. Cummins et al. (1991b: 1841)
77. Several other medical interventions—particularly in oncology—have similarly low survival rates, but because those interventions do not require the enrollment of an entire population, they do not seem to lead to CPR's "statisticulation": Huff (1954). And, of course, it is not because other "accepted" medical interventions are also problematic that we should not question CPR's survival rates. Ultimately, it is up to each of us to decide whether a 1–3 percent survival rate is low or high. The promoters of CPR would like you to believe that this survival rate is high, because any survival is better than its alternative, which would be zero. I differ. When I think of the 112 people I observed during resuscitative efforts in my study, I do not think about the one person who ended up walking out of the hospital but of the 101 people who were carried out the back door and of the ten other people who were transported to the intensive-care unit, some of them absolutely motionless and some of them shaking wildly with convulsions. When I reflect on CPR's outcome, I imagine one person—the lone survivor—tending the graves of a cemetery row with ninety-nine headstones of those who did not make it.
78. The evidence here is necessarily anecdotal because I was unable to find any studies in which a population was asked about its knowledge of survival rates.
79. Diem, Lantos, and Tulsky (1996)

80. Dr. Ron Walls, chairman of emergency medicine at Brigham and Women's Hospital, was quoted in the *Boston Globe* on June 12, 1996, as saying: "Even if TV shows make CPR look too easy or too successful, they're still educating the public about the value of CPR, and that is a very good thing."

81. Baer (1996)

82. Murphy et al. (1994)

83. Ibid., 548.

84. Murphy et al. (1994); Schonwetter et al. (1994)

85. Pasquale et al. (1996)

86. Ronco et al. (1995)

87. Ebell and Kruse (1994)

88. Vrtis (1992)

89. Lee, Angus, and Abramson (1996)

90. U.S. Department of Health and Human Services (1998)

91. Ebell and Kruse (1994)

92. U.S. Department of Commerce (1997)

93. Murphy and Finucane (1993)

94. Pasquale et al. (1996)

95. Anspach (1993: 170–75)

96. Eisenberg, Cummins, and Larsen (1991)

97. Hedges (1993: 42)

98. Ginsburg (1998)

CHAPTER 4

1. The three vignettes used in this chapter are composites of a number of observed resuscitative efforts in the emergency departments.

2. For a detailed ethno-methodological analysis of 911 calls, see Whalen, Zimmerman, and Whalen (1988).

3. Davis-Floyd (1992: 14)

4. The idea that individuals have multiple identities is one of the cornerstones of symbolic interactionist thought. See Goffman (1959); McCall and Simmons (1963); Mead (1934); Stone (1962); Star (1991). Individuals have identities relating to many spheres of their lives, such as occupational, political, and familial identities. To Klapp (1969: 39), identity depends of three basic variables: 1) what a person thinks about him or herself introspectively; 2) what others attribute to the individual (the social identity); and 3) feelings validated when "real to me" and when shared with others. In this chapter, I will mainly deal with multiple "social" identities, or the identities that others attribute to individuals. These identities are not mere hypothetical attributions; rather, they are socially situated and link an individual with others because of some significant commonality. Thus, although people have multiple identities, the identities are not immutable. They are constantly being subjected to change and challenge and require support and validation. Identities become strongest when an individual accepts the same identity that others have of him or her: McCall and Simmons (1963).

5. Lock (1989: 19)

6. Scheper-Hughes and Lock (1987)

7. Sharp (1995)

8. Goffman (1971: 51)

9. American Heart Association (n.d.)

10. Brenner and Kauffman (1993)

11. Perry (1993)

12. Ibid.

13. Chandra (1993: 283)

14. Chameides and Hazinski (1997: 11–5)

15. Ibid.

16. Heckman (1992: 24)

17. Whether this intention will be achieved in practice is discussed in the next chapters.

18. Foucault (1977, 1978)

19. See Parsons (1975) on the "sick" role.

20. Abbott (1988)

21. Goffman (1961)

22. Turner (1967: 97) noted in this regard: "Liminal personae nearly always and everywhere are regarded as polluting to those who have never been 'inoculated' against them, through having been themselves initiated in the same state."

23. Dillard (1995: 12)

24. These standing orders have been modified in certain counties around the country: see Chapter 7.

25. I will discuss the exceptions in the next chapter.

26. I would be paged as well.

27. Hirschauer (1991)

28. Ibid., 290

29. Singleton and Michael (1993)

30. Strauss (1969)

31. Glaser and Strauss (1968)

32. All patients who die less than twenty-four hours after admittance must be seen by a coroner.

33. This is required for all sudden deaths in EDs.

34. Denzin (1989)

35. Lorde (1980: 46–47)

36. See Strauss et al. (1985); Charmaz (1991)

37. Goffman (1959)

38. Rosaldo (1984: 190)

39. Ibid., 184

40. It is important to note that although sudden death poses deep emotional and existential questions, these emotions are not universal: see Scheper-Hughes (1992).

41. CPR might keep the body more viable for organ donation. The opportunity for organ donation adds an economic and moral dimension to CPR that

I will not address. It is well known that organ procurers play into the complex guilt feelings after sudden death to persuade relatives to donate organs. For an analysis of this gift-of-life discourse, see Sharp (1995).

42. Moore and Myerhoff (1977: 17–18)

43. Nuland (1994)

44. Scheper-Hughes and Lock (1987: 34)

45. Cussins (1998)

46. To add insult to injury, the relatives and friends often become a new target for medicalization. Because they receive an important share of the messages conveyed during reviving attempts, relatives and friends are part of the medicalization process. Relatives are not just thought of as kinship extensions of the patient but also as potential patients. Their physical and emotional reactions to the sorrow need to be managed with drugs, as the suggestion of the social worker to offer the stepdaughters a tranquilizer illustrates. The staff considers certain displays of emotion appropriate, whereas others, especially anger, are considered disturbing and unfitting.

CHAPTER 5

1. Glaser and Strauss (1964); Sudnow (1967)

2. Sudnow (1967: 74)

3. Ibid., 105.

4. Bauman (1992: 145)

5. For other critiques of Sudnow, see Crane (1975) and Zussman (1992).

6. Bauman does not argue that resuscitative efforts are not decided based on patients' social worth any longer, but that the social discrimination has shifted from "primitive" technology to more advanced medical technology such as organ donation and the "electronic computerized gadgetry."

7. Timmermans (1995b)

8. Berg (1997)

9. Schwartz and Griffin (1986); Dowie and Elstein (1988)

10. CPR-ECC (1973)

11. Omnibus Budget Reconciliation Act of 1990 (OBRA-90), Pub. L., 101–508, 4206 and 4751 (Medicare and Medicaid, respectively), 42 U.S.C. 1395cc (a) (I) (Q), 1295mm © (8), 1395cc (f), 1396a (a) (58), and 1396a (w) (Supp. 1991).

12. Conrad (1992)

13. The paramedics and EMTs actually follow a process very similar to the one I will describe. For an excellent paper on this, see Hughes (1980).

14. Death is obvious when rigor mortis has set in, decapitation has occurred, the body is consumed by fire, or there is a massive head injury with parts missing.

15. Implied consent refers to "a situation involving an unconscious patient in which care is initiated under the premise that the patient would desire such care if he or she were conscious and able to make the decision": Bledsoe, Porter, and Shade (1994: 45).

16. Lynch (1984: 67)

17. American Heart Association (1994: 3-3)

18. Cummins et al. (1991b)

19. Hughes (1971)

20. Joslyn (1994)

21. Tillinghast et al. (1991)

22. Chu et al. (1998)

23. Brookoff et al. (1994)

24. Hallstrom et al. (1993)

25. Ibid., 247.

26. Herlitz et al. (1997)

27. When this comment was made, a technician replied that he hoped he would be shot in the back by a jealous 19-year-old husband.

28. Hughes (1988)

29. Muller (1992)

30. Gazelle (1998)

31. Coser (1959); Lieber (1991); Yoels and Clair (1995)

32. This practice is not as marginal as one would think. Major medical journals regularly publish articles about the ethical implications of practicing intubation and other techniques on the "newly dead": see Burns et al. (1994).

33. Opinions vary about the best time to die. In theory, there is twice as much staff at the turn of shifts, which might guarantee more attention. In practice, however, the old staff is often tired and unwilling to do overtime to write the notes for the resuscitative effort. The new staff has to take care of an entire ward of new patients whom they haven't met yet and are anxious to move to the hospital or send home.

34. This is the Munchausen by proxy phenomenon, in which a caretaker, usually a mother, creates signs of illness and even death in a baby to receive medical attention.

35. Iserson and Stocking (1993)

36. It is important to note that the nurse was wrong in this instance.

37. The physician told me this story six years after it happened. My original question was, "Can you give me an example of a resuscitative effort that left a big impression on you?"

38. Fine and Asch (1988); Jones (1984); Mairs (1996); Zola (1984)

39. Hauswald and Tanberg (1993)

40. During one observation, a physician entertained the resuscitation team with a story of how he had once declared a patient deceased and, when everyone was leaving, he saw the chest moving rhythmically. They reconnected the patient, told the family about the unexpected improvement, and saw, to their surprise, that the patient started unassisted breathing. That patient lived for three days in the intensive-care unit. After that, the patient died from system failure and seizures.

41. There is also some evidence from other research that having an advance directive is in itself related to age, sex, race, socioeconomic status, and education. Schonwetter et al. (1994), for example, found a strong significant relationship between socioeconomic status and the desire for CPR.

42. Bauman (1992: 160)
43. Mulkay and Ernst (1991)
44. This is the original sense in which Goffman (1961) first introduced social death.
45. Mitchell and Snyder (1997); Morris (1990); Swain et al. (1993)

CHAPTER 6

1. When analyzing the different characteristics of work practices, Everett Hughes first drew attention to the difference between "routine" and "emergency" work. An "emergency" means here that special accommodations need to be worked out in order to make sense of an event. These accommodations might take a variety of forms, such as technical, institutional, cultural, or psychological adjustments. Routine work suggests that no such special accommodation is necessary and that the event can be handled without much change in the existing work practices. Hughes (1971: 316) wrote: "one man's routine of work is made up of the emergencies of other people."

2. Categorization is a nominal activity: the categories are not necessarily factual, but they are definitions developed by the staff of a particular situation. These definitions emerge collectively from practice and experience, and they reflect on practice. The process of categorizing ED patients has been extensively reported in the early medical sociology literature: See Dingwall and Murray (1983); Jeffery (1979); Hughes (1980); Roth (1972). Coming from a symbolic-interactionist–labeling perspective, Julius Roth (1972) explained categorization in terms of the social worth of the patient. Jeffery (1979) observed categorization of patients in three accident departments in England. He argued that the staff distinguish between "good" patients and "rubbish" (or crocks). Good patients tested the general competence and maturity of staff, while rubbish constituted trivia, drunks, overdoses, and tramps. Although the categorization of patients inevitably has moral overtones (some patients are preferred to others), in this chapter, I will analyze categorization as a means of understanding how emergency medical staff cope with resuscitative efforts in a routine-like manner. The assignment of different resuscitative efforts into categories is viewed as a way to come to terms with intervening in the gray area between life and death.

3. This is the name of one of the most popular resuscitation mannequins, whch is manufactured by the Danish Laerdal company.

4. Hughes (1971: 401)

5. Denzin (1989)

6. Some respondents remarked that during the last revision of the ACLS and CPR protocols, there seemed to be a greater acceptance of the limits of resuscitation technology. The protocols more explicitly indicated when resuscitative care was sufficient. In previous revisions, this issue was left to the discretion of physicians. Physicians also told me that they ran shorter resuscitative efforts compared with those they ran a decade ago. It is thus important to keep in mind that resuscitation technology is not a stable entity to which the staff

adapt over their career. As is shown in previous chapters, the technology itself changes over time and prompts change.

7. Stelling and Bucher (1973)

8. Benner (1984)

9. Geertz (1973)

10. Douglas (1992)

11. Anspach (1993)

12. See Hughes (1988).

13. See Benner (1984); Hughes (1988); Timmermans and Berg (1997).

14. Assuming that this was the way things always were, I remember thinking: "how am I ever going to be able to write a Ph.D. dissertation out of such a mess?"

15. American Heart Association (1994: 1–9).

16. Sudnow (1967)

17. See also Glaser and Strauss (1964); Kastenbaum and Aisenberg (1972); Lasagna (1973); Lowther (1988); Sudnow (1967); and Roth (1972).

18. Tye (1997)

19. Actually, I was forbidden by the IRB of one hospital to ask questions about this.

20. Thanatomimesis occurs when an organism initially appears to be dead but, on subsequent observation, proves to be alive: see Kastenbaum (1998).

21. Timmermans (1993), Chambliss (1996)

22. Quint (1966)

23. Sweeting and Gilhooly (1992)

24. Corr (1992)

25. Fox and Lief (1963: 13)

26. Elias (1984: 23)

CHAPTER 7

1. Eisenberg (1997: 252)

2. Safar and Bircher (1988: 383)

3. Star (1991: 53)

4. Gazelle (1998)

5. Hauswald and Tanberg (1993)

6. In an article "A Public Health Approach to Emergency Medicine: Preparing for the Twenty-first Century," the authors do not even mention CPR and ACLS. They see "alcohol, tobacco, and other drug abuse; injury; violence; sexually transmitted diseases and human immunodeficiency virus infection; occupational and environmental exposures; and the unmet health needs of minorities and women" as the main priorities: Bernstein et al. (1994: 277).

7. Beck and Leighninger (1959); Cummins quoted in Eisenberg (1997: 251)

8. Children are more likely to be resuscitated because of trauma than for a simple heart attack or stroke. A resuscitative effort is more likely to be medically justifiable in their situation; thus, the problem of indiscriminate resuscitative care

for children is not as widespread as for adults. I also think that it makes the most sense to make advanced cardiac care optional and not basic CPR. Basic CPR still has many positive communal characteristics. As I explain later, I am an advocate of more realistic information about what happens during CPR and what the chances are of reversing a sudden death.

9. Because listing all possible contingencies is impossible, a simple resuscitation will could have two choices: advanced resuscitative care under all circumstances or advanced CPR at the discretion of the professional health-care provider in charge.

10. Murphy et al. (1994)

11. I interviewed fifteen emergency–health-care providers in Belgium. Because of some structural differences in the emergency system and legislation, their experiences are only used as background experiences in this book.

12. Grint and Woolgar (1995)

13. To continue the truth-in-CPR campaign, it should also be pointed out in CPR courses that resuscitating is often smelly and messy. Good CPR requires that ribs break. Several of my respondents commented how eerie it is to feel ribs crack and then, with every compression, to sense how the edges of the broken ribs touch. Also, patients may throw up while you are doing mouth-to-mouth ventilation.

14. In some states programs exist for paramedics to verify quickly that a patient has a living will reflecting current wishes not to be resuscitated (Knox 1997). In Massachusetts, the program "Comfort Care" is administered via physicians and offers a wristband to people that states their wishes not to be resuscitated. It is too early to see whether this program has made a significant difference in the overuse of resuscitating. I observed one resuscitative effort in which the patient wore a typical silver health-care wristband stating that he was diabetic. It was only at the end of the reviving attempt that somebody noticed the wristband.

15. A possible solution is to send an EMT or paramedic trained in social work or trauma counseling.

16. Delooz (1993: 3)

17. Several books in any community library offer sample forms to draft a living will and a durable power of attorney for health care, and lawyers can, of course, help you, as well. To maximize the effects of these documents, give copies to your physician, lawyer, relatives, friends, clergy, and any others who might be involved in decision making about your dying.

18. Juhl (1997)

19. Personal conversation with emergency staff. For a discussion of this directive in a medical journal, see Iserson (1992).

20. Doyle et al. (1987)

21. See, for example, the recent debate in the *British Medical Journal* (Adams [1994]; Schilling, Crisci, and Judkins [1994]) or the ongoing debate in the *Journal for Emergency Nursing* (Martin [1991]; Osuagwu [1992, 1993]; Cox [1993]; Hanson and Strawser [1992]; Keating [1993]; Williams [1993]).

22. Timmermans (1994)

23. Cox (1993); Back and Rooke (1994); Grandstrom (1989)
24. Hanson and Strawser (1992: 104). Italics in original.
25. Post (1989)
26. Post (1989: 45–46)
27. Doyle et al. (1987); Post (1989); Hanson and Strawser (1992)
28. Reese (1994)
29. Goldman (1988)
30. Hanson and Strawser (1992: 106)
31. Williams (1993)
32. Hanson and Strawser (1992: 105)
33. Doyle et al. (1987)
34. Hanson and Strawser (1992: 106)
35. Renzi-Brown (1989)
36. Guzzeta and Mitchell (1997)
37. Cummins et al. (1991b)
38. Reese (1994)
39. I am grateful to Dessima Williams for making this point.
40. See Wertz and Wertz (1989: chap. 6); Starr (1982).
41. See Wertz and Wertz (1989: chap. 8). For an example of how Kübler-Ross's stage theory has become a normative expectation, see Timmermans (1991).

Appendix

1. See Timmermans (1991, 1993, 1994).
2. Latour (1987)
3. See Timmermans (1998b, 1999).
4. On the problems with one of those IRBs, see Timmermans (1995b).
5. Spradley (1980).
6. Glaser and Strauss (1967); Strauss and Corbin (1990).

References

Abbott, A. 1988. *The System of Professions: An Essay on the Division of Expert Labor.* Chicago: University of Chicago Press.

Adams, S. 1994. "Should Relatives Be Allowed to Watch Resuscitation?" *British Medical Journal* 308 (June 25): 1687–89.

Adgey, A. J., M. E. Scott, J. D. Allen, P. G. Nelsom, J. S. Geddes, S. A. Zaidi, and J. F. Pantridge. 1969. "Management of Ventricular Fibrillation Outside Hospital." *The Lancet* 1 (June 14): 1169–71.

American Heart Association. 1994. *Textbook of Advanced Cardiac Life Support* (3rd ed.). Dallas, Tex.: American Heart Association.

———. n.d. *Basic Life Support: Instructor's Manual.* Dallas, Tex.: American Heart Association.

Anspach, R. R. 1993. *Deciding Who Lives: Fateful Choices in the Intensive-Care Nursery.* Berkeley, Calif.: University of California Press.

Ariès, P. 1977. *The Hour of Our Death.* London: Allen Lane.

———.1976. *Western Attitudes Toward Death.* London, New York: Marion Boyars.

Back, D., and V. Rooke. 1994. "The Presence of Relatives in the Resuscitation Room." *Nursing Times* 90 (30): 34–35.

Baer, N. A. 1996. "Cardiopulmonary Resuscitation on Television: Exaggerations and Accusations." *New England Journal of Medicine* 334 (24): 1604–1605.

Baringer, J. R., Salzman, E. W., Jones, W. A., and A. L. Friedlich. 1961. External Cardiac Massage. *New England Journal of Medicine,* 2: 62–65.

Barry, E. 1804. *A Sermon Preached in the Parish Church of Allhallow's Barking: For the National Institution of the Royal Humane Society.* London: Nichols.

Bauman, Z. 1992. *Mortality, Immortality and Other Life Strategies.* Stanford, Calif.: Stanford University Press.

Beck, C. S., and D. S. Leighninger. 1962. "Reversal of Death in Good Hearts. *Journal of Cardiovascular Surgery,* 1962, 357–75.

———. 1959. "Resuscitation for Cardiac Arrest." *Postgraduate Medicine* 259 (May): 516–27.

Becker, L. B. 1993. "Methodology in Cardiac Arrest Symposium." *Annals of Emergency Medicine* 22 (1): 1–2.

Becker, L. B., B. H. Han, P. M. Meyer, F. A. Wright, K. V. Rhodes, D. W. Smith, and J. Barrett. 1993. "Racial Differences in the Incidence of Cardiac Arrest and Subsequent Survival." *New England Journal of Medicine* 329: 600–606.

Becker, L., B. M. P. Ostrander, J. Barrett, and G. T. Kondos. 1991. "Outcome of CPR in a Large Metropolitan Area: Where Are the Survivors?" *Annals of Emergency Medicine* 20: 355–61.

Benner, P. 1984. *From Novice to Expert: Excellence and Power in Clinical Nursing Practice*. Menlo Park, Calif.: Addison-Wesley Publishing.

Benoliel, J. Q. 1987. "Institutional Dying: A Convergence of Cultural Values, Technology, and Social Organization." In *Dying: Facing the Facts*, ed. H. Wass, F. H. Berardo, and R. A. Neimeyer. Washington, D.C.: Hemisphere Publishing.

Benson, D. W. 1961. "Recent Advances in Emergency Resuscitation." *Maryland State Medical Journal* 36 (August): 398–411.

Berek, K., P. Lechleitner, G. Luef, S. Felber, I. Saltuari, A. Schinnerl, C. Traweger, F. Dienstl, and F. Aichner. 1995. "Early Determination of Neurological Outcome After Prehospital Cardiopulmonary Resuscitation." *Stroke* 26 (4): 543–49.

Berg, M. 1997. *Rationalizing Medical Work: A Study of Decision Support Techniques and Medical Practices*. Cambridge, Mass.: MIT Press.

Berger, A. S. 1993. *Dying and Death in Law and Medicine: A Forensic Primer for Health and Legal Professionals*. Westport, Conn.: Praeger.

Bernstein, E., A. L. Kellerman, S. W. Hargarten, S. S. Fish, C. Flores, S. Krishel, T. D. Kirsch, S. R. Lowenstein, E. J. Mueller-Orsay, and D. P. Sklar. 1994. "A Public Health Approach to Emergency Medicine: Preparing for the Twenty-first Century." *Academic Emergency Medicine* 1 (3): 277–86.

Bledsoe, B. E., R. S. Porter, and B. R. Shade. 1994. *Paramedic Emergency Care*, 2nd ed. Englewood Cliffs, N.J.: Brady.

Bossaert, L., R. Vanhoweyweghen, and Group CRS. 1989. "Bystander Cardiopulmonary Resuscitaition in Out-of-Hospital Cardiac Arrest." *Resuscitation* (17): s55–s69.

Bourgeois, D., and B. van Heerikhuizen. 1980. "Een Interview met Philippe Ariès." In *Gestalten van de Dood*, ed. G. A. Back and L. Brunt. Baarn: Ambo.

Bowker, G. 1994. *Science on the Run: Information Management and Industrial Geophysics at Schlumberger, 1920–1940*. Cambridge, Mass.: MIT Press.

Bradwell, S. 1633. *Helps for Suddain Accidents Endangering Life*. London: n.p.

Brenner, B. E., and J. Kauffman. 1993. "Reluctance of Internists and Medical Nurses to Perform Mouth-to-Mouth Resuscitation." *Archives of Internal Medicine* 153: 1763–69.

Brookoff, D., A. L. Kellermann, B. B. Hackman, G. Somes, and P. Dobyns. 1994. "Do Blacks Get Bystander Cardiopulmonary Resuscitation as Often as Whites?" *Annals of Emergency Medicine* 24: 1147–50.

Burns, J. P., F. E. Reardon, and R. D. Truogh. 1994. "Using Newly Deceased Patients to Practice Resuscitation Procedures." *New England Journal of Medicine* 319: 439–41.

Bury, M. 1997. *Health and Illness in a Changing Society*. London and New York: Routledge.

Callahan, D. 1993. *The Troubled Dream of Life: Living with Mortality*. New York: Simon and Schuster.

Campbell, T. 1979. "Do Death Attitudes of Nurses and Physicians Differ?" *Omega* 9 (4): 43–49.

Cassell, E. 1976. "Dying in a Technological Society." In *Death Inside Out*, ed. P. Steinfels and R. Veatch. New York: Harper and Row.

Chambliss, D. F. *Beyond Caring: Hospitals, Nurses, and the Social Organization of Ethics*. Chicago: University of Chicago Press.

Chameides, L., and M. F. Hazinski. 1997. *Pediatric Advanced Life Support*. Dallas, Tex.: American Heart Association.

Chandra, N. C. 1993. "Mechanisms of Blood Flow During CPR." *Annals of Emergency Medicine* 22 (2): 281–88.

Charmaz, K. 1991. *Good Days, Bad Days: The Self in Chronic Illness and Time*. New Brunswick, N.J.: Rutgers University Press.

Chu, K., R. Swor, R. Jackson, R. Domeier, E. Sadler, E. Basse, H. Zaleznak, and J. Gitlin. 1998. "Race and Survival After Out of Hospital Cardiac Arrest in a Suburban Community." *Annals of Emergency Medicine* 31 (4): 478–82.

Clark, D. T. 1962. "Complications Following Closed-Chest Cardiac Massage." *Journal of the American Medical Association* 181 (4): 337–38.

Clarke, A. 1998. *Disciplinary Reproduction*. Berkeley, Calif.: University of California Press.

Clarke, A., and J. Fujimura. 1992. *The Right Tools for the Job*. Princeton, N.J.: Princeton University Press.

Collins, H. M. 1983. *Changing Order: Replication and Induction in Practice*. London: Sage.

Comroe, J. H., Jr. 1979a. "Retrospectroscope. '... In Comes the Good Air.' Part I: Rise and Fall of the Schafer Method." *American Review of Respiratory Disease* 119 (3): 803–809.

———. 1979b. "Retrospectroscope. '... In Comes the Good Air.' Part II: Mouth-to-Mouth Method." *American Review of Respiratory Disease* 119: 1025–1031.

———. 1979c. Retrospectroscope.'... In Comes the Good Air.' Part III: There Will Always Be an England." *American Review of Respiratory Disease* 120: 457–60.

Conrad, P. 1992. "Medicalization and Social Control." *Annual Review of Sociology* 18: 209–32.

Cooper, D. Y. 1975. "Minireview: Mouth-to-Mouth Resuscitation: Influence of Alcohol on Revival of an Old Technique." *Life Sciences* 16: 487–500.

Corr, C. A. 1993. "Coping with Dying: Lessons That We Should and Should Not Learn from the Work of Elisabeth Kübler-Ross." *Death Studies*, 17 (1): 69–83.

———. 1992. "A Task-Based Approach to Coping with Dying." *Omega* 24 (2): 81–94.

Coser, R. L. 1959. "Some Social Functions of Laughter." *Human Relations* 12: 171–82.

Cox, C. 1993. "Families and Codes—One Emergency Department's Experience (Letter)." *Journal of Emergency Nursing* (February): 5.

CPR-ECC. 1973. "Standards for Cardiopulmonary Resuscitation and Emergency Cardiac Care." *Journal of the American Medical Association* 227 (7): 836–68.

Crane, D. 1975. *The Sanctity of Social Life*. New York: Russell Sage.

Crawley, M., J. A. Lewis, and G. E. Ailshie. 1975. "Mobile Emergency Care Units." *Advances in Cardiology* 15: 9–24.

Cummins, R. O. 1995. "CPR and Ventricular Fibrillation: Lasts Longer, Ends Better." *Annals of Emergency Medicine* 25: 833–36.

———. 1993. "The Ustein Style for Uniform Reporting of Data from Out-of-Hospital Cardiac Arrest." *Annals of Emergency Medicine* 22 (1): 37–40.

Cummins, R. O., D. A. Chamberlain, N. S. Abramson, M. Allen, P. J. Baskett, K. Becker, T. L. Bossaert, H. K. Delooz, W. L. Dick, and M. Eisenberg. 1991a. "Recommended Guidelines for Uniform Reporting of Data from Out-of-Hospital Cardiac Arrest: The Utstein Style." *Circulation* 84 (2): 960–75.

Cummins, R., J. P. Ornato, and W. H. Thies. 1991b. "Improving Survival from Sudden Cardiac Arrest: The 'Chain of Survival' Concept." *Circulation* 83: 1832–47.

Cussins, C. 1998. "Ontological Choreography: Agency for Women in an Infertility Clinic." In *Differences in Medicine: Unraveling Practices, Techniques and Bodies*, ed. M. Berg and A. Mol. Durham, N.D.: Duke University Press, 164–201.

Davis-Floyd, R. 1992. *Birth as an American Rite of Passage*. Berkeley, Calif.: University of California Press.

de Beauvoir, S. 1965. *A Very Easy Death*. New York: Pantheon Books.

Delooz, H. H. 1993. *Standing Orders. Trainingsboek voor MUG Verpleegkundigen*. Leuven: KUL.

Demos, N. J., and S. M. Poticha. 1963. "Gastric Rupture Occurring During External Cardiac Resuscitation." *Surgery* 55 (3): 364–66.

Dempsey, D. 1975. *The Way We Die: An Investigation of Death and Dying in America Today*. New York: MacMillan Publishing.

Denzin, N. K. 1989. *Interpretive Interactionism*. Newbury Park, Calif.: SAGE Publications.

Diem, S. J, J. D. Lantos, and J. A. Tulsky. 1996. "Cardiopulmonary Resuscitation on Television." *New England Journal of Medicine* 334: 1578–82.

Dill, D. B., 1958. "Symposium on Mouth-to-Mouth Resuscitation." *Journal of the American Medical Association* 167 (3): 317–19.

———. 1951. "Manual Artificial Respiration." *U.S. Armed Forces Medical Journal* 3 (2): 171–84.

Dillard, J. 1995. "A Doctor's Dilemma." *Newsweek* (June 12), 13.

Dingwall, R., and T. Murray. 1983. "Categorization in Accident Departments: 'Good' Patients, 'Bad' Patients and 'Children.'" *Sociology of Health and Illness* 5 (2): 127–48.

Douglas, M. 1992. "Rightness of Categories." In *How Classification Works Among the Social Sciences*, ed. M. Douglas, N. Goodman, and D. Hull. Edinburgh: Edinburgh University Press, 239–72.

Dowie, J., and A. Elstein. 1988. *Professional Judgment: A Reader in Clinical Decision Making*. Cambridge: Cambridge University Press.

Doyle, C. J., H. Post, R. Burney, J. Maino, J. Keefe, and K. J. Rhee. 1987. "Family Participation During Resuscitation: An Option." *Annals of Emergency Medicine* 16 (6): 673–75.

Drinker, C. K., 1945. *Pulmonary Edema and Inflammation*. Cambridge, Mass.: Harvard University Press.

Ebell, M. H., and J. A. Kruse. 1994. "A Proposed Model for the Cost of Cardiopulmonary Resuscitation." *Medical Care* 32 (6): 640–49.

Editorial. 1965. "The Closed-Chest Method of Cardiopulmonary Resuscitation–Revised Statement." *Circulation* 31: 641–43.

———. 1962. "The Closed Chest Method of Cardiopulmonary Resuscitation: Benefits and Hazards." *Circulation* 26: 324.

Eisenberg, M. S. 1997. *Life in the Balance: Emergency Medicine and the Quest to Reverse Sudden Death.* New York: Oxford University Press.

———. 1992. "The Perfect Resuscitation." *Annals of Emergency Medicine* 21 (9), 1122–23.

Eisenberg, M. S., M. K. Copass, A. P. Hallstrom, B. Blake, C. Bergner, F. A. Short, and A. C. Cobb. 1980. "Treatment of Out-of-Hospital Cardiac Arrest with Rapid Defibrillation by Emergency Medical Technicians." *New England Journal of Medicine,* 302 (25): 1379–83.

Eisenberg, M. S., R. O. Cummins, S. Damen, M. P. Larsen, and T. R. Hearne. 1990b. "Survival Rates from Out-of-Hospital Cardiac Arrest: Recommendations for Uniform Definitions and Data to Report." *Annals of Emergency Medicine* 19 (1): 1249–59.

Eisenberg, M. S., R. O. Cummins, and M. P. Larsen. 1991. "Numerators, Denominators, and Survival Rates: Reporting Survival from Out-of-Hospital Cardiac Arrest." *American Journal of Emergency Medicine* 9 (6): 544–46.

Eisenberg, M., B. Horwood, R. Cummins, R. Reynolds-Haertle, and T. R. Hearne. 1990a. "Cardiac Arrest and Resuscitation: A Tale of 29 Cities." *Annals of Emergency Medicine* 19 (2): 179–86.

Elam, J. O. 1975. "Rediscovery of Expired Air Methods for Emergency Ventilation. In *Advances in Cardiopulmonary Resuscitation,* ed. P. Safar. New York: Springer-Verlag, 263–65.

Elam, J. O., E. S. Brown, and J. D. Elder. 1954. "Artificial Respiration by Mouth-to-Mask Method." *New England Journal of Medicine* 250 (18): 749–54.

Elam, J. O., D. G. Green, E. S. Brown, and J. A. Clements. 1958. "Oxygen and Carbon Dioxide Exchange and Energy Cost of Expired Air Resuscitation." *Journal of the American Medical Association* 167 (3): 328–34.

Elias, N. 1984. *De Eenzaamheid van Stervenden in Onze Tijd.* Amsterdam: Meulenhoff.

Epstein, S. 1996. *Impure Science: AIDS, Activism, and the Politics of Knowledge.* Berkeley: University of California Press.

Erhardt, C. L., and J. E. Berlin. 1974. *Mortality and Morbidity in the United States.* Cambridge, Mass.: Harvard University Press.

Feifel, H. 1959. *The Meaning of Death.* New York: McGraw-Hill.

Fine, M., and A. Asch. 1988. "Disability Beyond Stigma: Social Interaction, Discrimination, and Activism." *Journal of Social Issues* 44: 3–21.

Fletcher, J. 1977. "Elective Death." In *Understanding Death and Dying: An Interdisciplinary Approach,* ed. R. Fulton. New York: McGraw-Hill.

Fothergill, A. 1795. *An New Inquiry into the Suspension of Vital Action, in Cases of Drowning and Suffocation. Being an Attempt to Concentrate into a more Luminous Point of View, the Scattered Rays of Science, Respecting that Interesting though Mysterious Subject. To Elucidate the Proximate Cause, to Appreciate the Present Remedies, and to Point out the Best Method of Restoring Animation.* Bath: S. Hazard.

Foucault, M. 1978. *The History of Sexuality: An Introduction—Volume 1.* New York: Vintage Books.

———. 1977. *Discipline and Punish.* New York: Random House.

———. 1963. *Birth of the Clinic.* New York: Random House.

Fox, R. C. 1981. "The Sting of Death in American Society." *The Social Service Review*, 55 (1): 42–49.

———., ed. 1979. "The Social Meaning of Death." *The Annals of the American Academy of Political and Social Sciences*, 447.

Fox, R. C., and H. I. Lief. 1963. "Training for Detached Concern in Medical Students." In *The Psychological Basis of Medical Practice*, ed. H. I. Lief. New York: Harper and Row, 12–15.

Freud, S. 1918. *Reflections on War and Death*. New York: Moffat, Yard.

Fulton, R. 1977. *Death, Grief, and Bereavement: A Bibliography 1845–1975*. New York: Arno Press.

Gabriel, T. 1991. "A Fight to the Death: Was Ann Humphry's 'Final Exit' Intended to Pull the Plug on Her Ex-Husband's Right-to-Die Movement?" *New York Times* (December 8), 6, 46.

Gallagher, J. E., G. Lombardi, and P. Gennis. 1995. "Effectiveness of Bystander Cardiopulmonary Resuscitation and Survival Following Out-of-Hospital Cardiac Arrest." *Journal of the American Medical Association* 274 (24): 1922–25.

Gazelle, G. 1998. "The Slow Code: Should Anyone Rush to Its Defense?" *New England Journal of Medicine* 338 (7): 467–69.

Geertz, C. 1973. "Thick Description: Towards an Interpretive Theory of Culture." In *Interpretation of Cultures: Selected Essays*, C. Geertz. New York: Basic Books, 3–33.

Ginsburg, W. 1998. "Prepare to Be Shocked: The Evolving Standard of Care in Treating Sudden Cardiac Arrest." *American Journal of Emergency Medicine* 16 (3): 315–19.

Glaser, B. G., and A. L. Strauss. 1968. *Time for Dying*. Chicago: Aldine Publishing.

———. 1967. *The Discovery of Grounded Theory*. New York: Aldine de Gruyter.

———. 1965. *Awareness of Dying*. Chicago: Aldine Publishing.

———. 1964. "The Social Loss of Dying Patients." *American Journal of Nursing* 64: 119–21.

Goffman, E. 1971. *Relations in Public*. New York: Harper Colophon Books.

———. 1961. *Asylums: Essays on the Social Situation of Mental Patients and Other Inmates*. New York: Doubleday Anchor.

———. 1959. *The Presentation of Self in Everyday Life*. Garden City, N.Y.: Anchor Doubleday.

Goldman, B. 1988. "May I Watch? It May Become a More Common Question for MDs." *Canadian Medical Association Journal* (July 15): 148–49.

Gordon, A. S. 1967. "A History of Cardiopulmonary Resuscitation." In *Cardiopulmonary Resuscitation Conference Proceedings*, NRC-NAC, Washington,D.C. (May 23, 1966), 3–26.

Gordon, A. S., C. W. Freye, L. Gittelson, M. S. Sadove, and E. J. Beattie. 1958. "Mouth-to-Mouth Versus Manual Artificial Respiration for Children and Adults." *Journal of the American Medical Association* 167 (3): 320–27.

Gordon, A. S., M. S. Sadove, F. Raymon, and A. C. Ivy. 1951, "Critical Survey of Manual Artificial Respiration." *Journal of the American Medical Association* 147 (15): 1444–53.

Gorer, G. 1965. *Death, Grief, and Mourning*. Garden City, N.Y.: Doubleday.

Grace, W. J., and J. A. Chadbourn. 1969. "The Mobile Coronary Care Unit." *Diseases of the Chest* 55: 452–55.

Grandstrom, D. 1989. "The Family Has a Role Even During a Code." *RN* (August): 15–19.

Graves, J. R., A. Bang, A. Axelsson, M. Holmberg, K. Sonnerhagen, L. Ekstrom, J. Linqvist, and S. Holmberg. 1997. "Survival of Out-of-Hosptial Cardiac Arest: Their Prognosis, Longevity, and Functional Status." *Resuscitation* 35 (2): 117–21.

Gray, W., R. Capone, and A. Most. 1991. "Unsuccessful Emergency Medical Resuscitation: Are Continued Efforts Justified?" *New England Journal of Medicine* 325 (20): 1390–99.

Greene, D. G., R. O. Bauer, C. D. Janney, and J. E. Elam. 1956. "Crossed Ventilation in Apneic Patients. I. Blood Gas Changes." *American Journal of Physiology* 187: 602.

Grint, K., and S. Woolgar. 1995. *Deus ex Machina: Technology, Work, and Society.* Cambridge: Polity.

Guzzetta, C. E., and T. G. Mitchell. 1997. "Response to: High Touch in High Tech: The Presence of Relatives and Friends During Resuscitative Efforts." *Scholarly Inquiry for Nursing Practice* 11 (2): 169–173.

Hall, M. 1857. *Prone and Postural Respiration in Drowning.* London.

Haller, J. S. 1990. "The Beginnings of Urban Ambulance Service in the United States and England." *Journal of Emergency Medicine* 8: 743–55.

Hallstrom, A., P. Boutin, L. Cobb, and E. Johnson. 1993. "Socioeconomic Status and Prediction of Ventricular Fibrillation Survival." *American Journal of Public Health* 83: 245–48.

Hamilton, M., and H. Reid. 1990. *A Hospice Handbook: A New Way to Care for the Dying.* Grand Rapids, Mich.: William B. Eerdmans.

Hanson, C., and D. Strawser. 1992. "Family Presence During Cardiopulmonary Resuscitation: Foote Hospital Emergency Department's Nine-Year Perspective." *Journal of Emergency Nursing* 18 (2): 104–106.

Haraway, D. J. 1997. *Modest_Witness@Second_Millenium. FemaleMan_Meets_Oncomouse.* New York: Routledge.

Hauswald, M., and D. Tanberg. 1993. "Out-of-Hospital Resuscitation Preferences of Emergency Health Care Workers." *American Journal of Emergency Medicine* 11: 221–24.

Hawes, W. 1793. "Transactions of the Royal Humane Society." *Transactions of the Royal Humane Society*, London: n.p., i.

———. 1783. *An Address to the King and Parliament of Great-Britain, on Preserving the Lives of the Inhabitants to which are now added, Observations on the General Bills of Mortality.* London: J. Dodsley.

———. 1778. *An Address to the Public.* London: n.p.

Haynes, B. E., A. Mendoza, M. McNeil, J. Schroeder, and D.R. Smiley. 1991. "A Statewide Early Defibrillation Initiative Including Laypersons and Outcome Reporting." *Journal of the American Medical Association* 266 (4): 545–47.

Heckman, J. D. 1992. *Emergency Care and Transportation of the Sick and Injured*, 5th ed. n.p.: American Academy of Orthopaedic Surgeons.

Hedges, J. R. 1993. "Beyond Utstein: Implementation of a Multisource Uniform Data Base for Prehospital Cardiac Arrest Research." *Annals of Emergency Medicine* 22 (1): 41–46.

Herlitz, J., L. Elstrom, A. Axelsson, A. Bang, B. Wennerblom, L. Waagstein, M. Dellborg, and S. Holmberg. 1997. "Continuation of CPR on Admission to Emergency Department After Out-of-Hospital Cardiac Arrest: Occurrence, Characteristics, and Outcome." *Resuscitation* 33 (3): 223–31.

Hirschauer, S. 1991. "The Manufacture of Bodies in Surgery." *Social Studies of Science* 21: 279–319.

Huff, D. 1954. *How to Lie with Statistics.* New York: Norton.

Hughes, D. 1988. "When Nurse Knows Best: Some Aspects of Nurse–Doctor Interaction in a Casualty Department." *Sociology of Health and Illness* 10 (1): 1–22.

———. 1980. "The Ambulance Journey as an Information Generating Process." *Sociology of Health and Illness* 2 (2): 115–32.

Hughes, E. C. 1971. *The Sociological Eye: Selected Papers.* Chicago: Aldine Publishing.

Humphry, D. 1991. *Final Exit.* Eugene, Ore.: Hemlock Society.

———. 1978. *Jean's Way.* New York: Quartet Books.

Illich, I. 1976. *Medical Nemesis.* London: Calder and Boyars.

Iserson, J. 1992. "The 'No-Code' Tattoo—An Ethical Dilemma." *Western Journal of Medicine* 156 (3): 309–12.

Iserson, K. V., and C. Stocking, 1993. "Standards and Limits: Emergency Physicians' Attitude Toward Prehospital Resuscitation." *American Journal of Emergency Medicine* 11 (6): 592–94.

Jeffery, F. 1979. "Normal Rubbish: Deviant Patients in Casualty Departments." *Sociology of Health and Illness* 2 (2): 115–32.

Johns, R. J., and D. Y. Cooper. 1957. *Chemical Corps Medical Laboratory Report No. 761.* Edgewood, Md.: Army Chemical Center.

Jones, E. E. 1984. *Social Stigma: The Psychology of Marked Relationships.* New York: Freeman.

Joslyn, S. A. 1994. "Case Definition in Survival Studies of Out-of-Hospital Cardiac Arrest." *American Journal of Emergency Medicine* 12: 299–301.

Jude, J. R., W. B. Kouwenhoven, and G.G. Knickerbocker. 1964. "External Cardiac Resuscitation." *Monographs in the Surgical Sciences* 1: 59–119.

———. 1961a. "Cardiac Arrest: Report of Application of External Cardiac Massage on 118 Patients." *Journal of the American Medical Association* 178 (11): 1063–70.

———. 1961b. "A New Approach to Cardiac Resuscitation." *Annals of Surgery* 154 (3): 311–17.

Jude, J. R., J. Scherlis, and F. Farr. 1961. *Cardiopulmonary Resuscitation.* Baltimore: Maryland Heart Association.

Juhl, M. H. 1997. "A Tattoo in Time." *Newsweek* (October 13), 19.

Karpovich, P. V. 1953. *Adventures in Artificial Respiration.* New York: Association Press.

Kastenbaum, R. 1998. *Death, Society, and Human Experience.* Boston: Allyn and Bacon.

———. 1993. "Avery D. Weisman: An Omega Interview." *Omega* 27: 263–70.

Kastenbaum, R., and R. Aisenberg. 1972. *The Psychology of Death*. New York: Springer Publishing.

Kastenbaum, R., and C. Normand. 1990. "Deathbed Scenes as Expected by the Young and Experienced by the Old." *Death Studies* 14: 201–18.

Kaufman, S. R. 1993. *The Healer's Tale: Transforming Medicine and Culture*. Madison: University of Wisconsin Press.

Keating, Y. 1993. "More on Family Presence During Resuscitation (Letter)." *Journal of Emergency Nursing* 19 (6): 477–78.

Keith, A. 1909. "The Hunterian Lectures on the Mechanism Underlying the Various Methods of Artificial Respiration Practiced Since the Foundation of the Royal Humane Society in 1774." *The Lancet* 1: 745–49, 825–28, 895–99.

Kellehaer, A. 1990. *Dying of Cancer: The Final Years of Life*. Chur and London: Harwood Academic Publishers.

Kellerman, A. L., B. B. Hackman, G. Somes, T. K. Kreth, L. Nail, and P. Dobyns. 1993. "Impact of First-Responder Defibrillation in an Urban Emergency Medical Services System." *Journal of the American Medical Association* 270 (14): 1708–13.

Kevles, D. 1995. *The Physicists: The History of a Scientific Community in Modern America*. Chicago: University of Chicago Press.

Kevorkian, J. 1991. *Prescription Medicide*. Buffalo, N.Y.: Prometheus.

Killien, S. Y., J. P. Geyman, J. B. Gossom, and D. Gimlett. 1996. "Out-of-Hospital Cardiac Arrest in a Rural Area: A 16-Year Experience with Lessons Learned and National Comparisons." *Annals of Emergency Medicine* 28 (3): 294–99.

Killip, T. 1968. "Coronary Care Units: Current Policies and Results." In *Acute Myocardial Infarction*, ed. D. G. Julian and M. F. Oliver. Baltimore: Williams and Wilkins, 23–28.

Klapp, O. E. 1969. *Collective Search for Identity*. New York: Holt, Rinehart, Winston.

Klassen, G. A., C. Broadhurst, D. I. Peretz, and A. L. Johnson, 1963. Cardiac Resuscitation in 126 Medical Patients Using External Cardiac Massage. *The Lancet*, June: 1290–1292.

Kouwenhoven, W. B. 1966. "The Gray Area." *Industrial Medicine and Surgery* 25 (April): 271–74.

Kouwenhoven, W. B., J. R. Jude, and G. G. Knickerbocker. 1960. "Closed Chest Cardiac Massage." *Journal of the American Medical Association* 173: 1064–67.

Knox, R. 1997. Dying Wishes. *The Boston Globe*, (December 15) C1.

Kübler-Ross, E. 1969. *On Death and Dying*. New York: Macmillan.

Laborde, J. -V. 1894. *Les Tractions Rhytmées de la Langue: Moyen Rationnel et puissant de Raminer la Fonction Respiratoire et la Vie*. Paris: Germer Bailière.

Lasagna, L. 1973. "Physicians' Behavior Toward the Dying Patient." In *The Dying Patient*, ed. O. Brim, H. Freeman, and S. Levine. New York: Russell Sage Foundation, 83–101.

Latour, B. 1993. *We Have Never Been Modern*. Cambridge, Mass.: Harvard University Press.

———. 1987. *Science in Action: How to Follow Scientists and Engineers Through Society*. Cambridge, Mass.: Harvard University Press.

Lattin, D. 1997. "Expert on Death Faces Her Own Death: Kübler-Ross Now Questions Her Life's Work." *San Francisco Chronicle* (May 31), A1.

Lee, K. H., D. C. Angus, and N. S. Abramson. 1996. "Cardiopulmonary Resuscitation: What Cost to Cheat Death?" *Critical Care Medicine* 24 (12): 2046–52.

Leighninger, D. S. 1975. "Contributions of Claude Beck." In *Advances*, ed. Safar, 259–63.

Lieber, D. 1991. "Laughter and Humor in Critical Care." *Dimensions of Critical Care Nursing* 5: 162–70.

Lind, B., and J. Stovner. 1963. "Mouth-to-Mouth Resuscitation in Norway." *Journal of the American Medical Association* 185 (12): 933–35.

Liss, H. P. 1986. "A History of Resuscitation." *Annals of Emergency Medicine* 15: 65–72.

Lock, M. 1989. "Reaching Consensus About Death: Heart Transplants and Cultural Identity in Japan." *Society–Société* 13 (1): 15–26.

Lofland, L. 1975. *Toward a Sociology of Death and Dying.* Beverly Hills, Calif.: Sage Publications.

Lombardi, G., J. Gallagher, and P. Gennis. 1994. "Outcome of Out-of-Hospital Cardiac Arrest in New York City: The Pre-Hospital Arrest Survival Evaluation Study." *Journal of the American Medical Association* 271 (9): 682.

Lorde, A. 1980. *The Cancer Journals.* San Francisco: Aunt Lute.

Lowther, C. 1988. "Terminal Care in the Old." In *A Safer Death*, ed. A. Gilmore and S. Gilmore. New York: Plenum, 47–61.

Lynch, M. 1984. "'Turning Up Signs' in Neurobehavioral Diagnosis." *Symbolic Interaction* 7 (1): 67–76.

Mairs, N. 1996. *Waist-High in the World: A Life Among the Nondisabled.* Boston: Beacon Press.

Mannes, M. 1973. *Last Rights: A Case for the Good Death.* New York: Signet.

Martens, P., and O. Vanhaute. 1994. "Utstein Style Cardiopulmonary–Cerebral Resuscitation Registry for Out-of-Hospital Cardiac Arrest Between 1991 and 1993." The Belgian CPCR Study Group. *European Journal of Emergency Medicine* 1 (3): 115–19.

Martin, J. 1991. "Rethinking Traditional Thoughts (Letter)." *Journal of Emergency Nursing* 17 (2): 67.

McCall, G. J., and J. L. Simmons. 1963. *Identities and Interactions.* New York: Free Press.

Mead, G. H. 1934. *Mind, Self and Society.* Chicago: University of Chicago Press.

Miller, R. J. 1992. "Hospice Care as an Alternative to Euthanasia." *Law, Medicine, and Health* 20: 127–32.

Miranda, D. R. 1994. "Quality of Life After Cardiopulmonary Resuscitation." *Chest* 106 (2): 524–29.

Mitchell, D. T., and S. L. Snyder. 1997. *The Body and Physical Difference: Discourses of Disability.* Ann Arbor: University of Michigan Press.

Mitford, J. 1963. *The American Way of Death.* New York: Simon and Schuster.

Moller, D. W. 1990. *On Death Without Dignity: The Human Impact of Technological Dying.* New York: Baywood Publishing.

Moore, S. F., and B. Myerhoff. 1977. *Secular Ritual.* Assen–Amsterdam: Van Gorcum.

Mor, V. 1987. *Hospice Care Systems.* New York: Springer Publishing.

Morgan, R. R. 1961. "Laceration of the Liver from Closed-Chest Cardiac Massage." *New England Journal of Medicine* 265 (2): 82–83.

Morris, J. 1990. *Pride Against Prejudice: A Personal Politics of Disability.* London: Women's Press.

Mulkay, M., and J. Ernst. 1991. "The Changing Position of Social Death." *European Journal of Sociology* 32: 172–96.

Muller, J. H. 1992. "Shades of Blue: The Negotiation of Limited Codes by Medical Residents." *Social Science and Medicine* 34 (8): 885–98.

Munley, A. 1983. *The Hospice Alternative: A New Context for Death and Dying.* New York: Basic Books.

Murphy, D. J., D. Burrows, S. Santilli, A. W. Kemp, S. Tenner, B. Kreling, and J. Teno. 1994. "The Influence of the Probability of Survival on Patients' Preferences Regarding Cardiopulmonary Resuscitation." *New England Journal of Medicine* 330 (8): 545–49.

Murphy, D. J., and T. E. Finucane. 1993. "New Do-Not-Resuscitate Policies." *Archives of Internal Medicine* 153: 1641–48.

Myerhoff, B. 1978. *Number Our Days.* New York: Simon and Schuster.

Nagel, E. L., J. C. Hirschman, S. R. Nussenfeld, D. Rankin, and E. Lundblad. 1970. "Telemetry–Medical Command in Coronary Care and Other Mobile Emergency Care Systems." *Journal of the American Medical Association* 214: 332–38.

Niemann, J. T. 1993. "Study Design in Cardiac Arrest Research: Moving from the Laboratory to the Clinical Population." *Annals of Emergency Medicine* 22: 8–9.

NRC-NAC. 1966. *Cardiopulmonary Resuscitation Conference Proceedings.*

Nuland, S. B. 1994. *How We Die: Reflections on Life's Final Chapter.* New York: Albert A. Knopf.

Olson, D. W., J. LaRochelle, D. Fark, C. Aprahamian, T. P. Aufderheide, J. R. Mateer, K. M. Hargarten, and H. A. Stueven. 1989. "EMT Defibrillation: The Wisconsin Experience." *Annals of Emergency Medicine* 18 (8): 806–11.

Osuagwu, C. 1993. "More on Family Presence During Resuscitation (Letter)." *Journal of Emergency Nursing* 19 (4): 276–77.

———. 1992. "ED Codes: Keep the Family Out (Letter)." *Journal of Emergency Nursing* 17 (4): 363.

Pantridge, J. F., and J. S. Geddes. 1967. "A Mobile Intensive Care Unit in the Management of Myocardial Infarction." *The Lancet* 2: 270–72.

Paradis, L. F. 1985. *Hospice Handbook: A Guide for Managers and Planners.* Rockville, Md.: Aspen Publications.

Parsons, T. 1975. "The Sick Role and Role of Physician Reconsidered." *Millbank Memorial Fund Quarterly* 53: 257–78.

Pasquale, M. D., M. Rhodes, M. D. Cipolle, T. Hanley, and T. Wasser. 1996. "Defining 'Dead on Arrival': Impact on a Level I Trauma Center." *Journal of Trauma* 41 (4): 726–30.

Perry, M. 1993. "The Dilemma of a Good Samaritan." *Newsweek* (August 23), 11.

Pepe, P. E., N. S. Abramson, and C. G. Brown. 1994. "ACLS—Does it Really Work?" *Annals of Emergency Medicine* 23: 1037–41.

Pickering, A. 1995. *The Mangle of Practice: Time, Agency, and Science.* Chicago: University of Chicago Press.

Post, H. 1989. "Letting a Family in During a Code." *Nursing* (March): 43–46.

Quill, T. E. 1996. *Midwife Through the Dying Process.* Baltimore: Johns Hopkins University Press.

———. 1993. *Death and Dignity.* New York: Free Press.

———. 1991. "Death and Dignity: A Case of Individualized Decision Making." *New England Journal of Medicine* 325 (9): 658–60.

Quint, J. C. 1966. "Obstacles for Helping the Dying." *American Journal of Nursing* 66: 1568–71.

Reese, V. 1994. "Her Husband Was Dying and She Wanted to Watch the Code." *Nursing* (April): 32S–V.

Renzi-Brown, J. 1989. "Legally, It Makes Good Sense." *Nursing* (March): 46.

Riesman, D. 1935. *The Story of Medicine in the Middle Ages.* New York: Hoeber.

Rinaldi, A., and M. C. Kearl. 1990. "The Hospice Farewell: Ideological Perspectives of Its Professional Practitioners." *Omega* 21 (4): 283–300.

Rogers, K. 1966. "You Can Restore Life." *Coronet,* April 12.

Ronco, R., W. King, D. L. Donley, and S. J. Tilden. 1995. "Outcome and Cost at a Children's Hospital Following Resuscitation for Out-of-Hospital Cardiopulmonary Arrest." *Archives of Pediatric and Adolescent Medicine* 149 (2): 210–14.

Rosaldo, R. 1984. "Grief and a Headhunter's Rage: On the Cultural Force of Emotions." In *Text, Play, and Story: The Construction and Reconstruction of Self and Society,* ed. Edward Bruner. Prospect Heights, Ill.: Waveland Press, 178–99.

Ross, B. D. 1945. "Five Year Survey of Methods for Artificial Respiration." *Journal of the American Medical Association* 129 (6): 443–47.

Roth, J. A. 1972. "Some Contingencies of the Moral Evaluation and Control of Clientele: The Case of the Hospital Emergency Service." *American Journal of Sociology* 77 (5): 839–55.

Royal Humane Society. 1809. *Annual Report.* London: n.s.

———. 1803. *Annual Report.* London: n.s.

Safar, P. 1993. Cerebral Resuscitation After Cardiac Arrest: Research Initiatives and Future Directions. *Annals of Emergency Medicine,* 22 (2): 324–350.

———. 1975a. *Advances in Cardiopulmonary Resuscitation.* New York: Springer-Verlag.

———. 1975b. "From Back-Pressure, Arm-Lift to Mouth-to-Mouth, Control of Airway and Beyond." In *Advances,* ed. Safar, 266–76.

———. 1959. "Failure of Manual Respiration." *Journal of Applied Physiology* 14: 84–88.

Safar, P., and N. G. Bircher. 1988. *Cardiopulmonary Cerebral Resuscitation.* London: W.B. Saunders.

Schafer, E. A. 1904. "Description of a Simple and Efficient Method of Performing Artificial Respiration in the Human Subject, especially in Cases of Drowning, to which is Appended Instructions for the Treatment of the Apparently Drowned." *Medical and Chirurgical Transactions of the Royal Medical-Surgical Society* 87: 609–23.

———. 1903. "The Relative Efficiency of Certain Methods of Performing Artificial Respiration in Man." *Proceedings of the Royal Society of Edinburgh* 87: 39–51.

Schechter, D. C. 1969. "Role of the Humane Societies in the History of Resuscitation." *Surgery, Gynecology, and Obstetrics* 129: 811.

Scheper-Hughes, N. 1992. *Death Without Weeping.* Berkeley, Calif.: University of California Press.

Scheper-Hughes, N., and M. Lock. 1987. "The Mindful Body. *Medical Anthropology* 1: 6–41.

Schilling, R. J., C. Crisci, and K. V. Judkins. 1994. "Should Relatives Watch Resuscitation? (Letters)." *British Medical Journal* 309 (August 6): 406–407.

Schonwetter, R. S., R. M. Walker, D. R. Kramer, and B. E. Robinson. 1994. "Socioeconomic Status and Resuscitation Preferences in the Elderly." *Journal of Applied Gerontology* 13 (2): 157–71.

Schwartz, S. and T. Griffin. 1986. *Medical Thinking—The Psychology of Medical Judgment and Decision Making.* New York: Springer Publishing.

Shapin, S., and S. Schaffer. 1985. *Leviathan and the Air-Pump: Hobbes, Boyle, and the Experimental Life.* Princeton, N.J.: Princeton University Press.

Sharp, L. A. 1995. "Organ Transplantation as a Transformation Experience: Anthropological Insights into the Restructuring of the Self." *Medical Anthropology Quarterly* 9 (3): 337–89.

Siebold, C. 1992. *The Hospice Movement: Easing Death's Pain.* New York: Twayne.

Silvester, H. R. 1858. *The True Physiological Method of Restoring Persons Apparently Drowned or Dead.* London.

Singleton, V. and M. Michael. 1993. "Actor–Networks and Ambivalence: General Practitioners in the UK Cervical Screening Programme." *Social Studies of Science* 23 (2): 227–65.

Sontag, S. 1978. *Illness as Metaphor.* New York: Farrar, Straus, and Giroux.

Spradley, J. P. 1980. *Participant Observation.* New York: Holt, Rinehart, and Winston.

Star, S. L. 1991. "Power, Technologies and the Phenomenology of Conventions: On Being Allergic to Onions." In *A Sociology of Monsters: Essays on Power, Technology and Domination,* ed. J. Law. London: Routledge.

———. 1989. *Regions of the Mind: Brain Research and the Quest for Scientific Certainty.* Stanford, Calif.: Stanford University Press.

Starr, P. 1982. *The Social Transformation of American Medicine.* New York: Basicbooks.

Stelling, J., and R. Bucher. 1973. "Vocabularies of Realism in Professional Socialization." *Social Science and Medicine* 7 (September): 661–75.

Stephenson, H. E., Jr. 1974. *Cardiac Arrest and Resuscitation.* St. Louis: CV Mosby.

Stevens, R. 1989. *In Sickness and Wealth: American Hospitals in the Twentieth Century.* New York: Basic Books.

Stoddard, S. 1978. *The Hospice Movement.* New York: Vintage.

Stone, G. P. 1962. "Appearance and the Self." In *Human Behavior and Social Processes,* ed. A. Rose. Boston: Houghton Mifflin, 86–118.

Strauss, A. 1969. *Mirrors and Masks: The Search for an Identity.* San Francisco: Sociology Press.

Strauss, A., and J. Corbin. 1990. *Basics of Qualitative Research*. Newbury Park, Calif.: Sage Publications.

Strauss, A., S. Fagerhaugh, B. Suczek, and C. Wiener. 1985. *Social Organization of Medical Work*. Chicago: University of Chicago Press.

Strive, R. 1803. "Annual Sermon." *British Critic*, 658–62.

Sudnow, D. 1967. *Passing On: The Social Organization of Dying*. Englewood Cliffs, N.J.: Prentice Hall.

Swain, J., V. Finkelstein, S. French, and M. Oliver. 1993. *Disabling Barriers–Enabling Environments*. London: Open University.

Sweeney, T. A., J. W. Runge, M. A. Gibbs, J. M. Raymond, R. W. Schafermeyer, H. J. Norton, and M. J. Boyle Whitesel. 1998. "EMT Defibrillation Does Not Increase Survival from Sudden Cardiac Death in a Two-Tiered Urban–Suburban EMS System." *Annals of Emergency Medicine* 31 (2): 234–40.

Sweeting, H. N., and M. L. Gilhooly. 1992. "Doctor, Am I Dead? A Review of Social Death in Modern Societies." *Omega* 24: 251–69.

Swor, R. A., R. E. Jackson, M. Cynar, E. Sadler, E. Basse, B. Boji, E. J. Rivera-Rivera, A. Maher, W. Grubb, R. Jacobson, and D. L. Dalbec. 1995. "Bystander CPR, Ventricular Fibrillation, and Survival in Witnessed, Unmonitored Out-of-Hospital Cardiac Arrest." *Annals of Emergency Medicine* 25 (6): 780–84.

Tang, W., M. H. Weil, R. B. Schock, S. Yoji, J. Lucas, S. Sun, and J. Bisera. 1997. "Phased Chest and Abdominal Compression–Decompression: A New Option for Cardiopulmonary Resuscitation." *Circulation* 95 (5): 1335–40.

Thompson, L. 1984. "Cultural and Institutional Restrictions on Dying Styles in a Technological Society." *Death Education* 8: 223–29.

Tillinghast, S., K. M. Doliszny, T. E. Kottke, O. Gomez-Marin, P. G. Lilja, and B. C. Campion. 1991. "Change in Survival from Out-of-Hospital Cardiac Arrest and Its Effect on Coronary Heart Disease Mortality." *American Journal of Epidemiology* 134: 851–61.

Timmermans, S. 1999. "Closed-Chest Cardiac Massage: The Emergence of a Discovery Trajectory." *Science, Technology and Human Values* 24 (2): 213—240.

———. 1998a. Social Death as a Self-Fulfilling Prophecy: David Sudnow's "Passing On" Revisited. *The Sociological Quarterly* 39 (3): 453—472.

———. 1998b. "Debating Universality: The Case of Closed-Chest Cardiac Massage." *International Journal of Sociology and Social Policy* 18 (5): 107–36.

———. 1997. High Tech in High Touch: The Presence of Relatives and Friends during Resuscitative Efforts. *Scholarly Inquiry for Nursing Practice,* 11 (2): 152–167.

———. 1996. Saving Lives or Identities? The Double Dynamic of Technoscientific Scripts. *Social Studies of Science,* 26. (4): 769–799.

———. 1995a. *Saving Lives: A Historical and Ethnographic Study of Resuscitation Techniques*. Ph.D. diss., University of Illinois, Champaign-Urbana.

———. 1995b. "Cui Bono? Ethnographic Research and Institutional Review Boards." *Studies in Symbolic Interaction* 19: 155–75.

———. 1994. "Dying of Awareness: The Theory of Awareness Contexts Revisited." *Sociology of Health and Illness* 16 (3): 322–36.

———. 1993. "The Paradox of Nursing Terminal Patients in a General Belgian Hospital." *Omega* 27 (4): 281–93.

———. 1991. "Stervensbegeleiding? Dat wordt hier niet gedaan." *Tijdschrift voor Sociologie* 12 (2): 1–20.

Timmermans, S., and M. Berg. 1997. "Standardization in Action: Achieving Local Universality Through Medical Protocols." *Social Studies of Science* 27 (2): 273–305.

Tisherman, S. A., K. Vandevelde, P. Safar, T. Morioka, W. Obrist, L. Corne, R. F. Buckman, S. Rubertsson, H. E. Stephenson, A. Grenvik, and R. J. White. 1997. "Future Directions for Resuscitation Research. V. Ultra-Advanced Life Support." *Resuscitation* 34: 281–93.

Turner, V. 1967. *The Forest of Symbols.* Ithaca, N.Y.: Cornell University Press.

Tye, L. 1997. "Doctor Had Little Hope of Success." *Boston Globe* (September 1), A6.

U.S. Department of Commerce. 1997. *Statistical Abstract of the U.S.* Washington, D.C.: U.S. Government Printing Office.

U.S. Department of Health and Human Services. 1998. *Health United States 1996–97 and Injury Chartbook.* Hyattsville, Md.: DHHS Publications.

Veatch, R. M. 1991. "Models for Ethical Medicine in a Revolutionary Age." In *Biomedical Ethics*, ed. T. A. Mappes and J. S. Zembaty. New York: McGraw-Hill.

Vesalius, A. 1543. *De Humani Corporis Fabrica: Libri Septem.* Oprinus: Basel.

Vrtis, M. C. 1992. "Cost/Benefit Analysis of Cardiopulmonary Resuscitation: A Comprehensive Study." *Nursing Management* 23: 44–51.

Waitzkin, H. 1979. "A Marxist Interpretation of the Growth and Development of Coronary Care Technology." *American Journal of Public Health* 69 (12): 1260–68.

Wald, F. S. 1996. "The Emergence of Hospice Care in the U.S." In *Facing Death: Where Culture, Religion, and Medicine Meet*, ed. Howard M. Spiro, Mary G. McCrea, and Lee Palmer Wandel. New Haven, Conn.: Yale University Press, 81–90.

Waters, R. M. 1943. "Simple Methods for Performing Artificial Respiration. *Journal of the American Medical Association* 123: 559–661.

Weaver, W. D. 1991. "Resuscitation Outside the Hospital—What's Lacking?" *New England Journal of Medicine* 325 (20): 1437–40.

Weil, M. H., and W. Tang. 1997. "Cardiopulmonary Resuscitation: A Promise as Yet Unfulfilled." *Disease-a-Month* 43 (7): 433–94.

Wertz, R. W., and D. C. Wertz. 1989. *Lying In: A History of Childbirth in America.* New Haven, Conn.: Yale University Press.

Whalen, J., D. H. Zimmerman, and M. R. Whalen. 1988. "When Words Fail: A Single Case Analysis." *Social Problems* 35 (4): 335–62.

Williams, M. 1993. "Family Presence During Resuscitation (Letter)." *Journal of Emergency Nursing* (December): 478–79.

Winchell, S. W., and P. Safar. 1966. "Teaching and Testing Lay and Paramedical Personnel in Cardiopulmonary Resuscitation." *Anesthesia and Analgesia* 45 (4): 441–49.

Yates, R. 1807. *A Sermon, Preached at the Anniversary of the Royal Humane Society.* London: J. Nichols and Son.

Yoels, W. C., and J. M. Clair. 1995. "Laughter in the Clinic: Humor as Social Organization." *Symbolic Interaction* 18 (1): 39–59.

Zola, I. K. 1984. *Missing Pieces: A Chronicle of Living with a Disability*. Philadelphia: Temple University Press.

Zussman, R. 1992. *Intensive Care*. Chicago: University of Chicago Press.

Index